Acknowledgements

Research, editorial, graphics and photography by  d-squared^{design}

Project team: Mark Hewitt, Clare Gerrard, Paul Saltmarsh

Project team at the DfES:

Mukund Patel	School Building and Design Unit (SBDU)
Lucy Watson	SBDU
Alison Wadsworth	SBDU
Susan Clarke	Vulnerable Children Team, SEN Division
Lorraine Morris	Vulnerable Children Team, SEN Division
Joanna Driscoll	Vulnerable Children Team, SEN Division

Members of the Steering Group:

Yvonne Hill	Headteacher of The Children's Hospital School at Great Ormond Street and University College London Hospital
Brian Goldsmith	Consultant Architect
Heather Frost	Independent Education Consultant (Children with Medical Needs)
Terry Waller	Education Officer: Inclusion & SEN, Becta
Mike Collin	Teacher in Charge, Hospital Home Teaching, Newham, LEA
June Lancaster	Clinical Adviser, NHS Estates

The DfES and NHS Estates would like to thank the following for their help in co-ordinating DfES and DoH documents:

Brian Coapes	Senior Procurement Manager, NHS Estates
Christine Humphrey	Child Health and Maternity Branch, DOH

The DfES and NHS Estates would also like to thank all the hospital school staff and pupils who helped in the collection of case study examples.

Contents

Foreword 1

Introduction 3
Vision 3
Scope 4
Context 4
Audience 4
Structure 5

Section A: Background and briefing 6
A1   Need 6
A2   Hospital provision 7
A3   Links to the home school 7
A4   Responsibilities and funding 7
A5   Consultation 8
A6   Teamworking 8
A7   Pupil profile 9
A7.1   Length of stay 9
A7.2   Age range 9
A7.3   Mobile pupils 9
A7.4   Non-mobile pupils 10
A7.5   Isolation cases 10
A7.6   Patients with mental health problems 11
A7.7   Pupils with special educational needs (SEN) 12
A7.8   Parents and siblings 12
A8   Staff 12
A8.1   Staff profile 12
A8.2   Collaboration with youth workers and play specialists 12
A8.3   Teacher–pupil ratio 13
A9   Curriculum 13
A9.1   Creative arts 14
A9.2   ICT 15
A9.3   Extra-curricular activities 16

Section B: Design guidance 17
B1   Planning 17
B1.1   Location 17
B1.2   The range of spaces 18
B1.3   Links between spaces 19
B1.4   Security and safety 20
B2   Teaching areas 20
B2.1   Classroom 22
B2.2   Satellite spaces 24
B2.3   Ward teaching 24
B2.4   Isolation teaching 25
B2.5   Facilities without dedicated classrooms 25
B3   Non-teaching areas 26
B3.1   Storage 26
B3.1.1   Teaching storage 26
B3.1.2   Administration storage 27
B3.1.3   Personal storage 27
B3.2   Entrance areas 27

B3.3   Administration office(s) 28
B3.4   Staff room 28
B3.5   Ancillary spaces 28
B3.6   Toilets 29
B3.7   Circulation 30
B4   Outside space 30
B4.1   Location 31
B4.2   Landscaping 32
B4.3   Equipment 32
B4.4   Shade 32
B4.5   Outdoor storage 33
B4.6   Outdoor security and safety 33
B5   Design of elements 33
B5.1   Materials and surfaces 33
B5.2   Floors 34
B5.3   Walls 34
B5.4   Ceilings 34
B5.5   Doors and windows 35
B5.6   Colour and texture 36
B6   Furniture and fittings 36
B6.1   Ergonomics 37
B6.2   Tables 38
B6.3   Benching/worktops 38
B6.4   Work surfaces for ICT 39
B6.5   Seating 39
B6.6   Display 40
B6.7   Storage furniture 40
B6.8   Trolleys 41
B6.9   Partitioning 42
B7   Environmental design and services 43
B7.1   Lighting 43
B71.1   Daylighting 43
B7.1.2 Electric light 44
B7.1.3 Glare and reflection 44
B7.1.4 Shading 45
B7.1.5 Visual impairment 46
B7.2   Power supply 46
B7.3   Educational technology 46
B7.4   Water 47
B7.5   Ventilation and heating 47
B7.6   Acoustics 48
B8   Designing for children and young people with mental health problems 49

Section C: Case studies 51
Case study 1: Suite of classrooms in a large children's and young people's hospital 52
Case study 2: Suite of classrooms in a specialist paediatric hospital 56
Case study 3: Single school room at a secondary referral hospital 60
Case study 4: Suite of classrooms with a satellite in a tertiary referral hospital 64
Case study 5: Young people's unit in a tertiary referral hospital 68
Case study 6: Psychiatric unit in a tertiary referral hospital 72
Case study 7: School attached to psychiatric unit for young people 76
Key to symbols 80

Glossary and acronyms 82
Index 84

Foreword

By the Parliamentary Under Secretary of State for Sure Start, Baroness Catherine Ashton,

and

The Minister of State for Social Care, Long term Care, Disability and Mental Health, Jacqui Smith.

This Government is committed to the provision of high quality education for pupils who are unable to attend school because of illness or injury.

As part of that commitment the DfES and the Department of Health issued, in November 2001, joint statutory guidance, **Access to Education for children and young people with Medical needs**. This set out minimum national standards of education for children who are unable to attend school because of medical needs, and recognised the important part that both health and education play in the well being of children and young people.

This new joint DfES/NHS Estates (an Agency of the Department of Health) guidance on **Meeting the educational needs of children and young people in hospital** is part of the Government's continuing commitment to raising standards of achievement and providing equal access to all, including those children and young people who cannot attend school because of their medical needs. It also supports the new health care National Service Framework for Children.

Collaborative working between Local Education Authorities, hospital trusts, and all those involved in hospital design and refurbishment, is vital in ensuring that children and young people have the best accommodation possible to ensure continuing access to high quality education.

We therefore commend this guidance to you, and trust that it will enable those involved in hospital design to develop innovative and appropriate solutions to the often complex challenges surrounding the education of children and young people in hospital settings.

Introduction

In November 2001, the DfES and the Department of Health jointly published new statutory guidance **Access to education for children and young people with Medical needs**. This sets out minimum national standards of education for children and young people who are unable to attend school because of their medical needs. The guidance contributes to the Government's strategy to promote equal access to education for all children and young people. It also forms part of a joint approach by the Department for Education and Skills and the Department of Health which recognises the important part that both health and education play in the wellbeing of children and young people.

This new guidance on education accommodation in hospital settings complements **Access to education for children and young people with Medical needs**[1] and will help to ensure that these children have the best possible education.

This guide is also designed to accompany and complement **Hospital accommodation for children and young people**[2]. It will supersede **Meeting the educational needs of children in hospital, Design Note 38**[3].

Readers of this guidance may also find **Access to Education for Children with Medical Needs - A Map of Best Practice**[4] a useful accompanying document.

This document is a joint publication by NHS Estates and DfES.

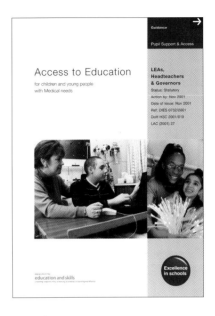

Vision

Education is a key ingredient in the recovery process and plays an important part in the hospital experience of children and young people by maintaining a sense of normality in the hospital environment. Education facilities in hospitals also play an important role in helping to maintain links between the pupil, home tuition and the mainstream school environments, thereby ensuring as much continuity of education as possible. Children and young people should have as much education as their medical condition allows so that they are able to continue their education and keep up with their studies.

Good design of the education environment in hospital can significantly enhance the delivery of learning. This guide is intended to help all stakeholders ask pertinent questions, consult successfully and develop imaginative and appropriate design solutions.

Notes

1 Department for Education and Skills/Department of Health. **Access to education for children and young people with Medical needs**. TSO, 2001. Ref. 0732/2001.

2 NHS Estates. **HBN 23: Hospital accommodation for children and young people**. TSO, 2003 (forthcoming).

3 Department of Education and Science. **Design Note 38: Meeting the educational needs of children in hospital**. DES, 1984. ISSN 0141-2825.

4 Peter Farrell and Karen Harris. **Access to Education for Children with Medical Needs - A Map of Best Practice**. Educational Support and Inclusion Research and Teaching Group, Faculty of Education, The University of Manchester. February 2003.

Scope

The aim of the guide is to assist the process of designing excellent education provision in hospitals, whether new or refurbished. Information from a survey of current best practice provides the foundation for the recommendations made. This information should be used by stakeholders to consult and inter-act thoroughly and effectively to ensure the best possible outcome for each particular case. Local conditions should be researched and understood completely, since the provision needed will vary greatly depending on the patient profile of each facility. This guidance is specifically focused on the educational environment in hospitals which has requirements deriving from the educational agenda.

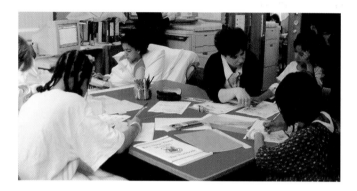

Key Stages 3 and 4 pupils in an education facility.

Context

This guide is written at a time when patterns of healthcare and education in hospitals are changing. Patients are spending less time in hospital and more time being cared for at home. By contrast, in some clinical areas such as mental health care, patients are tending to stay for longer periods and numbers are increasing. The delivery of education is changing due to the use of information and communications technology (ICT), allowing learning to take place in both a real and virtual education environment, which has a positive impact on educational facilities in hospitals.

Audience

The guide should help to ensure that primary care trusts, hospital trusts, local education authorities, governors and school staff can properly plan to provide the appropriate resources for the education facility. It will be useful to:
- local education authorities;
- project managers;
- hospital trust estates managers;
- estates consultants;
- architects;
- education facility heads and teachers;
- governors.

Structure

The guide is written in three sections:

Section A: Background and briefing gives the context for designing spaces for hospital education.

Section B: Design guidance sets out key issues for the design of spaces for hospital education.

Section C: Case studies examines seven different examples of education facilities in hospitals.

The guide does not present model solutions, or prescriptions, but through examining existing case studies analyses strengths and weaknesses and sets up a framework for alerting design teams to key issues.

Section A: Background and briefing

A1   Need

Section 19 of the 1996 Education Act states that Local Education Authorities (LEAs) must provide suitable education for school age children who cannot attend school because of medical needs. This includes provision while they are in hospital. Children should be taught the National Curriculum wherever possible and are entitled to as much education as their medical condition allows. The decision about when a child or young person should receive education should be made in conjunction with the medical staff and the patient. In cases of recurring illness, the child or young person is entitled to education from the first day of admission.

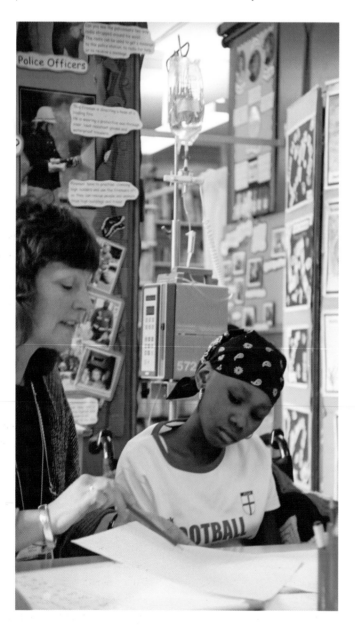

Pupil with a drip trolley attending a class in the schoolroom.

A2 Hospital provision

In the framework of healthcare planning, there is a move towards two types of hospital:

- a few large centres for tertiary referral[5];
- smaller, less specialised hospitals (for secondary referral).

There is a trend towards separating provision for young people and children, which recognises the different needs of the age groups. These variations are likely to lead to different functional and spatial demands. Thus, during the briefing process, it is essential that the specific requirements deriving from the particular patient profile of the location should be addressed.

Design teams should familiarise themselves with all relevant work delivered as part of the **Children's National Service Framework**[6] **(NSF)**, which will set out the key qualitative parameters for children and young people in hospital. NHS Estates' **Achieving Excellence Design Evaluation Toolkit** should also prove helpful as a general checklist of hospital design criteria[7].

A3 Links to the home school

Links between the home school and hospital school are important and must be properly established and catered for. Increasingly, electronic links are assisting the flow of information.

All education facilities in hospitals should keep daily records of the teaching provided to individual pupils. These records are important for keeping the home school informed of the educational progress of the pupil while in hospital. Similarly, home schools should provide speedy and up-to-date information on their pupils to the hospital education facility.

One of the key accommodation implications of this is the amount of administration storage space needed for records (see Section B3.1.2).

A4 Responsibilities and funding

The way in which accommodation is funded varies, as illustrated by the Case Studies. It is the responsibility of the LEA to fund the education and the hospital trust's duty to provide the accommodation. **Access to education** states:

> "Hospitals are required to provide for the accommodation needs of children and young people receiving education in hospital but may seek a contribution to the capital and running costs of this accommodation from the LEA. LEAs should collaborate closely with their respective health authorities [now Primary Care Trusts] to ensure the availability of suitable teaching and storage accommodation in hospitals."[8]

Notes

5   Primary care is with the GP; secondary referral is to a local hospital; and tertiary referral is where children are referred by their local hospitals for specialist treatment. Children coming to a tertiary referral unit will come from all over the country and overseas.

6   **The Children's National Service Framework.** The Government published the first part of the Children's National Service Framework in April 2003. This includes the **Standard for Hospital Services** and an **Emerging Findings** consultation document. The full Children's NSF will be published in 2004.

7   AEDET can be downloaded from the NHS Estates web site **http://www.nhsestates.gov.uk/ patient_environment/index.asp**

8   Department for Education and Skills/Department of Health. **Access to education for children and young people with Medical needs.** TSO, 2001. Ref. 0732/2001, p. 36, para. 8.15.

A5   Consultation

Clear and methodical consultation is vital[9]. In a hospital education facility, there are a number of different stakeholders and interested parties who should be consulted to ensure that all relevant inputs are gathered in the brief. These will include:

- head teacher, teaching and school staff, and governors;
- patients/pupils;
- key medical personnel (including senior nurses) involved in children's treatment and play staff;
- representatives of NHS Estates;
- representatives of the hospital trust estates and management teams;
- local education authorities;
- representatives of children's management teams.

It is recommended that everyone with an interest in the project, whether designing or briefing, visit at least one other good example of a hospital education facility guided by a teacher from the facility.

Research and consultation with primary and secondary level pupils will be essential to get a clear view of their learning experiences and needs. Consultation is a two way process, allowing the design team to acquire detailed knowledge of stakeholder preferences, and engaging the stakeholders actively in thinking about potential outcomes of the project. This is likely to lead to a more successful handover and occupation of the project on completion, since the stakeholders will feel fully involved with, and understand the constraints and opportunities of, the final accommodation.

In order to ensure that the gathering of view points and inputs is clearly documented, it is recommended that the design team prepares pro-forma questionnaires to gather information from each of the various stakeholders. This will ensure that later preparation of briefing documentation is based on measured inputs from the consultation process, and any changes to the brief can be discussed with reference to documented consultation. A good strategy is to send these questionnaires in advance of a meeting, since this allows the stakeholder time for thought, but face to face meetings are strongly recommended, since this format tends to allow more detailed, specific and nuanced consultation to occur.

A6   Teamworking

Good management of the relationship between clinical, educational and other key professional staff (such as youth workers and play specialists) plays a significant part in the achievement of the educational ambitions of a facility.

The consequences of a well structured teamworking policy were clearly evident in the Case Studies made during the preparation of this guidance. Facilities where teamworking is emphasised tend to share space (clinical and educational) more frequently. The benefits of this include the educational facility being able to occasionally use a larger area on the ward for events such as a drama workshop. The use of clinical space for occasional activities such as educational examinations can also be facilitated by good teamworking practice.

A meeting place which is large enough to contain the key cross-disciplinary professional staff (such as a staff room or medical or educational administration office) will encourage good teamworking practice.

Notes

9   A good example of a consultation process which contains some useful recommendations can be seen in the L4A report: **"Building the best" The new Derbyshire Children's Hospital.** Report of consultation workshops with staff, parents and children, 1990 (available from the Department of Health).

A7 Pupil profile

Access to education for children and young people with Medical needs states: "Most of the children for whom hospital schools or hospital teaching services provide are hospital in-patients, although a few chronically ill children may attend daily from home. Some may be admitted for only a few days, while others may remain on wards or in units for longer. Others may attend the hospital school regularly for a few days a week, returning home or to school for the rest of the week."[10] At the design stage it is important to establish what the particular profile of treatment the ward/hospital is offering, and whether there are particular accommodation requirements.

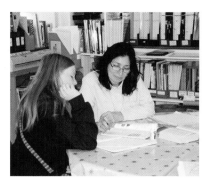

Pupil and member of staff in an educational facility.

A7.1 Length of stay

Young people's stays in hospital tend to be briefer now than in the past[11]. Due to advances in medical treatments, many children survive conditions which would previously have been fatal and as a consequence tend to have more special requirements. Patients with serious conditions also tend to spend long periods in hospital, but not always in one stay.

Patients with mental health problems tend to spend longer periods in hospital or purpose designed special units (frequently from six months upwards).

A7.2 Age range

Pupils referred for education in hospital include all ages (compulsory up to 16, and encouraged up to 19). Patients may be taught in any age group or separated into children and young people. This may reflect the teaching method of the education facility or the way wards are arranged (see Section A2). The needs of different age groups should be taken into account when designing the facility. For example, a young person preparing for an educational examination would need to spend more time in private study. In this case, smaller satellite teaching and study spaces are very important, particularly where there are likely to be groups of younger children in the main classroom areas.

A7.3 Mobile pupils

The number of pupils that are able to come to the schoolroom to learn will depend on the patient profile. Some will need additional space to accommodate vehicles or equipment that they use. Examples of pupils requiring extra space for equipment include:

- Orthopaedic[12] patients, who may be in wheelchairs[13] or on beds, and who may have limbs protruding beyond the wheelchair or bed (in plaster casts, for example).

[Handwritten notes in margin: freud, S / Hubbock / Justus, R / Little / NHS / Schaefor. / Mark, A, Barnes.]

Notes

10 Department for Education and Skills/Department of Health. **Access to education for children and young people with Medical needs**. HMSO, 2001. Ref. 0732/2001, p. 7, para. 1.9.

11 See R. MacFaul and U. Wernecke. **Recent trends in hospital use by children in England**. Archives of Disease in Childhood, Vol. 85, 2001, pp. 203-207.

12 Orthopaedic: relating to the correction of bone injuries or deformities.

13 See Brian C. Goldsmith. **Design data for wheelchair children**. The Disabled Living Foundation, 1979.

- Pupils who are weak as a result of treatment or their condition - also in wheelchairs.
- Patients who are attached to equipment (such as drip stands).
- In some cases, a pupil may also have a nurse in attendance.
- Pupils with a long term disability who may be in wheelchairs.

Pupils on oncology[14] wards will have a range of symptoms but most of them will need to be attached to mobile electronic equipment. Children undergoing chemotherapy are likely to vomit; thus, classrooms should have the appropriate equipment and facilities (such as gloves and containers) close to hand to deal with this situation. In addition, treatment may leave patients in a temporarily neutropaenic (immune-deficient) state.

A7.4   Non-mobile pupils

In some facilities, depending on the medical profiles of the pupils, teaching on the wards may absorb much of the teaching time.

Provision is needed for good bedside teaching and for teaching in isolation units (see A7.5). Ward and isolation teaching is resource intensive. Where a patient's mobility is restricted to one place on the ward, some teaching equipment and materials will need to be stored on the ward. For example, it would be preferable for the work plan and books of dialysis patients who come in regularly (often to the same ward) as day patients to be stored on the ward. Other resources will be brought from a central storeroom (see Section B3.1.1).

A7.5   Isolation cases

Some pupils will require isolation, barrier nursing[15] or reverse barrier nursing[16], all of which will have an effect on the accommodation requirements of the educational facility. In some cases, an additional classroom or resource base may be needed (even if the number of pupils does not warrant this) to allow the appropriate level of separation.

Neutropaenic or immune deficient patients cannot mix with others because they are vulnerable to infection. If these patients are well enough to leave the ward, a separate area should be provided in the school facility. Sometimes neutropaenic patients will need to be taught in isolation rooms on the ward, in which case teachers will need to take the appropriate level of protection (gowns and gloves) and material provision (disinfecting where necessary). Consideration should be given to providing storage for duplicate materials.

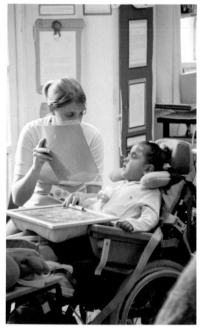

Pupil with limited mobility taking part in a class in the schoolroom with a specialist helper.

Notes

14 Oncology: relating to the treatment of cancer.

15 Barrier nursing: a patient nursed in isolation because of infection which may be contagious. Equipment for use with such patients must be disposable or washable and be thoroughly disinfected before being returned to normal use: See NHS Estates. **HFN 30: Infection control in the built environment**. TSO, 2002.

16 Reverse barrier nursing: patient nursed in isolation to prevent infection (for example, of an open wound, scald, burn). Equipment for use with such patients may be washed in disinfectant before being used, or may need to be new on each occasion.

Customer name: Robinson, Ellie . (Miss)
Customer ID: 0333598898

Title: Meeting the educational needs of children
and young people in hospital: a design guide

ID: 1703658138
Due: 5/2/2015,23:59

Title: Education and children with special
needs : from segregation to inclusion
ID: 1704311723
Due: 5/2/2015,23:59

Title: The education of children with medical
conditions
ID: 1702882873
Due: 5/2/2015,23:59

Total items: 3
2/01/2015 16:23
Checked out: 3
Overdue: 0
Hold requests: 5
Ready for pickup: 3

Need help? Why not Chat with Us 24/7?
See the Contact Us page on the library website:
library.leedsbeckett.ac.uk

A7.6 Patients with mental health problems

Patients with mental health problems are usually taught in school facilities[17] that are integral to the mental health unit or hospital in which they are being treated. However, they sometimes share educational facilities with other patients. Patients admitted to hospital with physical symptoms may later be found to have no organic evidence of illness, and the cause of their illness may then be attributed to psychological/psychosomatic difficulties. Their stay in hospital tends to be longer than patients with organic illness, which is due to the difficulty of diagnosis and to the problem of finding the most suitable treatment. A full curriculum may be accessed by patients with mental health problems and facilities for practical science and design and technology are needed for older pupils. This is particularly important, since patients may spend an average of four months in the inpatient unit[18] and therefore should be able to carry on the full range of subjects.

Creative arts such as painting and pottery also play a major role in developing emotional intelligence[19] and are very therapeutic activities. Facilities for these activities are therefore essential.

Children in psychiatric units should have access to some kind of PE facility. Younger pupils should have access to suitable play areas. Access to outside space, and access to transport for outings and trips to parks are also essential.

Security is of particular importance for classrooms accommodating patients with mental health problems. Some pupils may require a more than usually secure environment either to protect them or those around them. Some patients[20] with mental health problems may manifest sudden aggression or bouts of anti-social behaviour, which can be disruptive and frightening for other patients and potentially dangerous for themselves. In certain situations, this requires a teacher to pupil ratio of 1:4 or less, the presence of specialist nursing staff or the provision of a room for individual teaching.

Pupils will occasionally need to withdraw from the classroom; they should be able to do this quickly, causing the minimum disruption. The provision of a suitable space, which allows the pupil privacy, is essential. Some pupils will need to move to a larger space away from others.

All these requirements should be taken into account when sizing classrooms and designing accommodation as a whole for a school which is attended by patients with mental health problems. It is also important that the overall learning environment is calm, orderly and protective.

A summary of the key design issues related to patients with mental health problems is given in section B8.

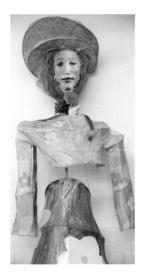

Life size puppet made by pupils at a school attached to a psychiatric unit.

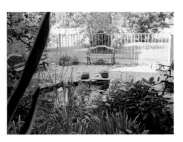

Garden and pond made by pupils at a school attached to a psychiatric unit.

"It is an important part of getting better that the environment is attractive and well looked after, and that there is some ownership of the environment by young people." Head of School in a Psychiatric Unit.

Notes

17 See NHS Estates. **Mental health facilities for children and young people**. TSO (forthcoming).

18 Report for this guidance from Janette Steel, Head of Child and Psychiatry Unit, BKWC Mental Health NHS Trust.

19 Report for this guidance from Janette Steel, Head of Child and Psychiatry Unit, BKWC Mental Health NHS Trust.

20 See Department for Education and Skills. **Promoting Children s Mental Health Within Early Years and School Settings**. DfES, 0112/2001.

A7.7   Pupils with special educational needs (SEN)[21]

There may be a significant number of pupils with special educational needs, including visual[22] and hearing difficulties. Guidance should be sought from the medical and teaching representatives on the client body of any particular requirements that the patients may have, but general notes on good design are included in Section B of this document.

Design teams should be aware of their responsibilities to ensure good design and access within the terms of the Disability Discrimination Act 1995 and the Disability Rights Commission (DRC) Act 1999[23]. Reference should also be made to the SEN (Special Educational Needs) Code of Practice[24].

A7.8   Parents and siblings

Families sometimes bring healthy siblings to the hospital, particularly to tertiary referral units which may be distant from home. These siblings may be catered for in the education facility, so this should be taken into account at the design stage. Parents, family, friends and carers will regularly visit the children on the wards and they will occasionally be present in the hospital schoolroom. Other adults such as nurses may also come into the schoolroom from time to time. These additional people should be taken into account when considering space provision.

A8   Staff

A8.1   Staff profile

The profile of hospital teaching is changing, from teachers with expertise in hospital education to a mix which includes teaching assistants. Teachers in hospitals have to be flexible about how, where and with what materials they teach to be able to deal with unconventional schoolroom conditions. It is also important that all back-up, administration, storage, service and support spaces are considered and well designed to give teachers optimum working conditions.

A8.2   Collaboration with youth workers and play specialists

A youth worker may be involved with young people's education (for example, focusing on developing independence skills and looking outwards towards work and career). Play specialists may also be present in the hospital (for example, helping children to talk about their anxieties during their stay in hospital). Close collaboration with the school staff is beneficial to an integrated provision; it is generally helpful if accommodation for the youth worker and play specialist is co-ordinated with the education

Notes

21 Refer also to
    http://www.doh.gov.uk/dda/index.htm

22 For useful general guidance on this
    subject, see Department for Education
    and Employment. **Building Bulletin
    90: Lighting design for schools.** TSO,
    1999.

23 Information is available from
    http://www.disability.gov.uk

24 The new edition of the **SEN Code** was
    published in December 2001 and came
    into effect from 1 January 2002:
    Department for Education and Skills.
    **Special Educational Needs: Code of
    Practice.** TSO, 2001. Ref. 581/2001.
    http://inclusion.ngfl.gov.uk

provision, so that maximum advantage can be taken of overlaps and joint activities. For many facilities, it is advisable to locate youth workers and play specialists close to the school accommodation.

A8.3 Teacher–pupil ratio

A teacher pupil ratio of 1:6 is common practice. For safety reasons, enclosed teaching rooms are preferred with a minimum of two staff members present (in case one of the teachers should have to leave the room, and to protect both pupils and teachers). When teaching pupils with mental health problems, a teacher pupil ratio of 1:4 or less is common.

When teaching at the bedside on the ward 1:1 teaching is possible because of the continual presence of nursing staff.

A9 Curriculum

Children being educated in hospital should have access to the full National Curriculum wherever possible[25]. However, flexibility is important and pupils' individual plans of work need to take into account their capabilities, which may alter during their stay.

PE, for example, might involve more gentle exercise and dance (exercising fine motor skills and social skills) compared with the more robust activities of a mainstream school PE programme.

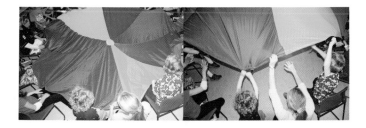

Practical activities such as chemistry experiments are limited by the lack of specialist facilities in a hospital, but hospital education facilities attempt to cover the full range of practical subjects as far as possible. In the future, virtual, online laboratories will facilitate practical science work for pupils.

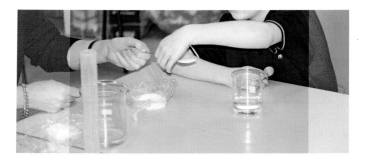

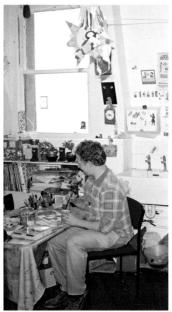

Play specialist in a childrens ward, located adjacent to the schoolroom.

"Our system of collaboration and mutual support with the Youth Workers and Activities Co-ordinators are an intrinsic part of the units philosophy of multi-disciplinary team work. We share spaces and ideas constructively." Head of School and teacher in an adolescent unit.

PE for Key Stages 1 and 2 pupils.

"PE is important, although it can look rather different to what you might conventionally expect, ballet dancing with feathers, for example." Head of a hospital school.

Science lesson in a shared Key Stage 1 and 2 classroom.

Notes

25 See Department for Education and Skills/Department of Health. **Access to education for children and young people with Medical needs**, 2001. Ref. 0732/2001, p. 30, para. 6.12.

Pupils may occasionally need to sit a public examination while in hospital and staff need to have access to a room that can provide suitable conditions (see Section B2.2).

Some facilities offer extra-curricular activities on weekday evenings. During half-term and long holidays, extra-curricular 'holiday schools' are often held.

A9.1   Creative arts

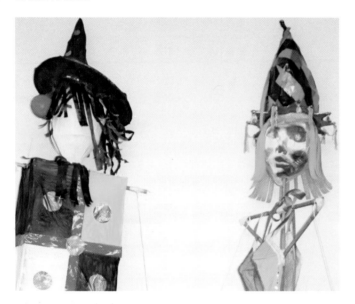

Life size puppets made by pupils at a school attached to a psychiatric unit.

The therapeutic and educational value of the creative arts is universally recognised[26] and in hospital education facilities it is of particular value[27]. Teachers may, for example, use artwork as a means to assist pupils to reflect on and understand their hospital experience. Education facilities often collaborate with art groups or professional art organisations to develop particularly ambitious art projects. This will have space implications (see Section B2.1).

It is important to ensure that there is adequate provision for storing art materials, which can be bulky. Paper, including large sheets, needs to be easily accessible. Craft materials are often heavy and need to be stored within easy and safe reach.

Drama, music work and performance are also highly valued in hospital facilities, and it is not uncommon for specialists, visiting actors and musicians to run workshops and deliver lessons as part of the general provision of activities. These sessions can be particularly valuable for less mobile pupils.

Drama and music may take place in small 'class' groups, or larger groups may be assembled for an occasional activity such as group singing or a performance. There may also be some individual music teaching. All these situations should be taken into account when designing the education facility. There needs to be storage for musical instruments both on and off the ward.

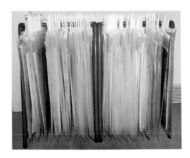

Flat artwork storage.

Notes

26 See NHS Estates. **The art of good health - using visual arts in healthcare**. TSO, 2002.

27 There is an increasing body of work citing the value of art in the hospital environment generally, and specific guidance on how to develop art projects as an integral part of the initial design and subsequent running of the hospital. See NHS Estates. **The art of good health – a practical handbook**. TSO, 2002.

A9.2 ICT

ICT has had a significant impact on the nature and scope of teaching both in the schoolroom and on the wards. It is of particular benefit in the following areas:

- isolation cases;
- special needs teaching;
- distance learning;
- continuing social contact with home and school;
- continuity with home school (work plans provided in web-based folders which can be accessed electronically from anywhere, allowing the work to 'follow' the pupil, whether they are at home, in hospital or in mainstream education);
- record-keeping (although this is currently mainly paper based).

Multiple educational benefits facilitated by ICT.

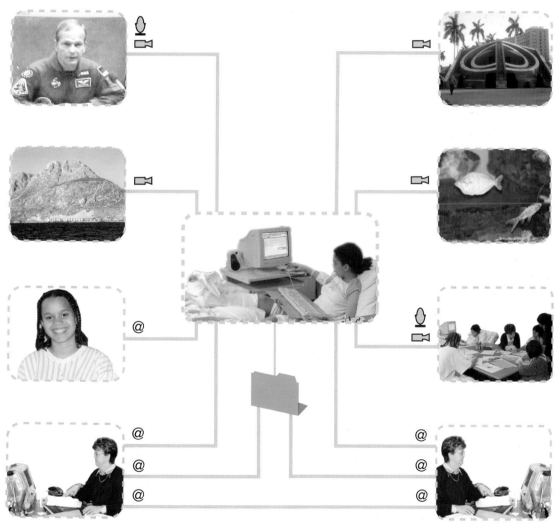

Home school teacher

Hospital school teacher

 Webcam

@ Email

Videoconferencing

Easy access to Internet services is important in a hospital education facility. They provide educational and social links for pupils and administrative links for staff. The Internet offers access to a huge range of appropriate educational material, and it is likely that online facilities will be used increasingly in education for the foreseeable future. Direct contact with home school teachers can be maintained through work and feedback on email. Social contact with friends can also be facilitated by email.

Continuity of work plans can be achieved by keeping them logged and updated in electronic form. Home schools, where appropriate, can provide input into these work plans.

Web-cams and video-conferencing are used already by some hospital education facilities to link students in real time to their home school classrooms and to link classrooms within a hospital. They are also used to link to other educational centres such as museums. Although currently this is used more frequently for maintaining social and community bonds, it is likely that in future such ICT capability will form an important part of the educational experience. A web-cam linked to a laptop or desktop work-station could be used either in a classroom or bed location. ICT facilities at a patient's bedside are improving rapidly, which helps teaching[28].

Electronic storage of all kinds of information is useful for reducing the amount of hard-copy storage required to keep educational facilities up-to-date with curriculum revision.

A9.3   Extra-curricular activities

A ward will be operational for 24 hours a day, normally seven days a week, whereas the schoolroom will usually be closed for holidays, weekends and most evenings. Some education facilities prefer to remain off limits for other activities to prevent damage or loss of resources. However, others allow teaching areas to be used for related activities (for example, youth workers or play specialists in the vacation periods).

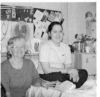

"If I could change anything, I would have a computer with email outside the resource room, as this is locked at 3.30pm each day and at weekends." Year 10 pupil.

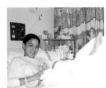

"I use the computers to write poems and stories, which is good because it helps to exercise my arm after an injection. I also work in bed on a clipboard." Year 8 pupil in a hospital school.

"I really enjoy videoconferencing. On one day I spoke to people in the U.S., Israel and Manchester from a small room." Secondary age pupil.

"Videoconferencing is not only used for 'lessons'. The Carol Service at Christmas was linked all around the hospital to children who could not physically make it to the chapel, as well as to a special school in Slough. They could not only watch the service but could interact by joining in the readings and songs." Hospital School ICT co-ordinator.

Notes

28 "Patient Power" is a strategy to bring telephones and televisions to each bed. More information is available on **http://www.nhsestates.gov.uk/patient_environment/index.asp**

Section B: Design guidance

B1   Planning

It is critical that planning the education facility begins at the early stages of planning the whole hospital project, whether it be a refurbishment or new build.

B1.1   Location

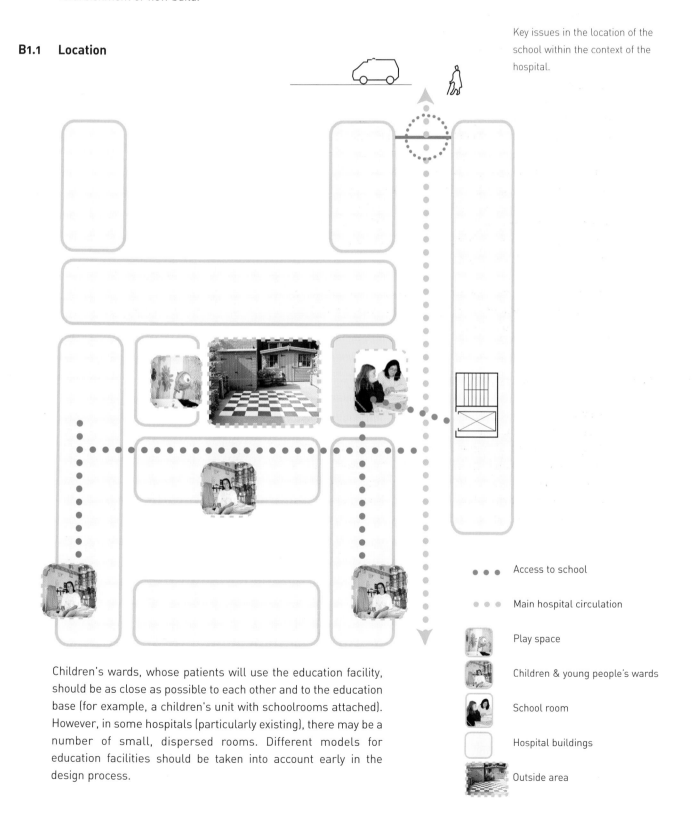

Key issues in the location of the school within the context of the hospital.

• • • Access to school

• • • Main hospital circulation

Play space

Children & young people's wards

School room

Hospital buildings

Outside area

Children's wards, whose patients will use the education facility, should be as close as possible to each other and to the education base (for example, a children's unit with schoolrooms attached). However, in some hospitals (particularly existing), there may be a number of small, dispersed rooms. Different models for education facilities should be taken into account early in the design process.

Any educational facility (whether dispersed or in a suite) should be on the same level as the children's wards. The distance between these wards and the school spaces should be minimised, reducing the amount of teachers' travelling time better spent with pupils and ensuring the maximum security for pupils.

Proximity is also good for the pupils, since it will allow them the greatest opportunity to enjoy the benefit of going to the schoolroom.

The education facility should be:
- highly visible in the layout of the hospital, so that staff, parents and pupils become aware of its presence and location;
- located near lifts with easy access to all children's treatment areas;
- easily accessible for beds (this applies equally to outside spaces).

In most of the Case Studies examined for the guidance, group visits and trips organised for the pupils were cited as an important part of the educational programme. The education facility should therefore be suitably located to allow easy access to a parking area for transportation.

B1.2   The range of spaces

Although the range of spaces varies, all dedicated education facilities in hospital have the following basic requirements:
- discrete, distinct classroom spaces for teaching;
- smaller 'satellite' teaching spaces which can be used as an academic examination room, interview room or for teaching immune-deficient pupils in the main facility, but outside of the wards;
- staff room;
- head teacher's office (where appropriate);
- administration office;
- good storage for teaching materials and equipment (a storeroom per class and a central storeroom);
- storage for the personal belongings of staff;
- WCs, separate for staff and pupils;
- a shower for staff (this could be part of the general staff area provision of the trust);
- ideally, an outside area for play and education.

The ratio of area of teaching to support for hospital education, from case study analysis, is optimally around 60% teaching to 40% support. Outside space is not counted in this calculation.

Potential range of spaces for an education facility

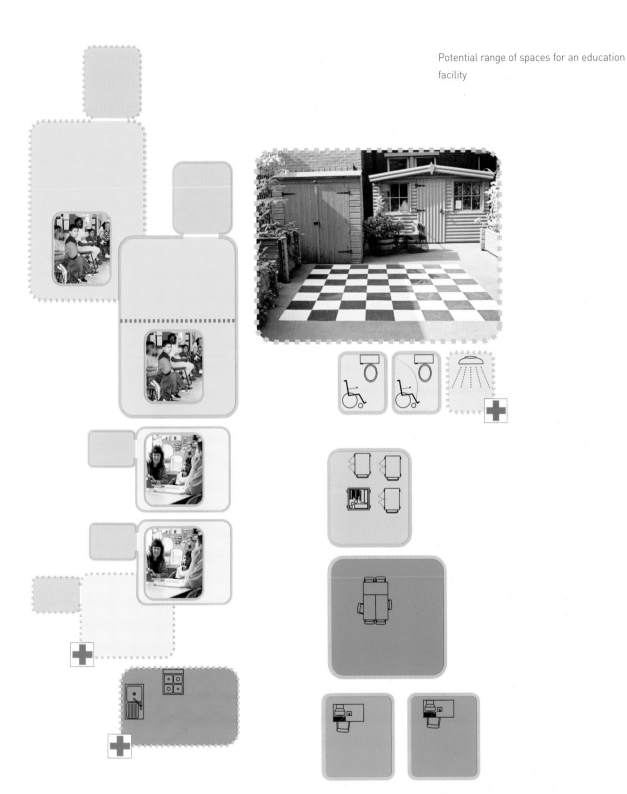

B1.3   Links between spaces

The main classroom(s), smaller satellite spaces and any outside space should be grouped as closely as possible. Links with other hospital areas that may house occasionally shared or group activities such as the social area of the ward will also need to be taken into account (see Case Study 4 where there is significant sharing between the school and ward areas). Playrooms should be near educational spaces.

Classroom
Satellite teaching space
Store
Kitchen
W.C.
Staff room
Head Teacher's office
Administration
May be NHS Trust provision
outside school boundary
Outside area

Provision for the parents close to the wards and school is an important planning issue for the design of the hospital. Although this will not fall within the brief for the education facility, a clear understanding of the relationship between the spaces for the family and the spaces for the education facility is recommended.

B1.4   Security and safety

There are two principal aspects to security:
- keeping control on who enters the educational facility to protect people and property;
- ensuring that pupils are not liable to wander unattended where this might put them at risk.

All spaces in an educational facility should be lockable, and all access points into and out of the facility should have controlled security. This will range from an attended reception to key, swipe or code operated locks. CCTV may be provided depending on the policy of the hospital trust.

Educational equipment, particularly laptop computers, peripherals, removable memory and drives are vulnerable. Hospital contents are almost impossible to insure; therefore, primary security (lockability) is vital. Visual supervision, possibly associated with a reception, should be considered.

Health and safety issues, particularly fire precautions and means of escape in case of fire, must be borne in mind when designing security arrangements. All escape routes must allow override on locks for means of escape in case of fire. Reference should be made to the relevant Building Regulations and NHS Estates Firecode guidance[29].

Access to equipment and space, particularly computer terminals for use of the Internet, may be needed after school hours, and ways to achieve this should be discussed at the planning stage.

Some pupils will be long-stay patients, and the facilities available in the education areas may be in demand for both study and recreational use. In case a pupil requires urgent medical attention, all teaching spaces and toilets should be equipped with a rapid communication alarm to a nursing station. The best solution is a nurse call to the ward area.

B2   Teaching areas

The particular profile of the educational facility should be established before deciding on teaching area requirements. Key questions such as whether children are taught separately from young people should be established as part of the information-gathering and briefing exercise (see Section A7). The kind of space provision, design of the layout, use and specification

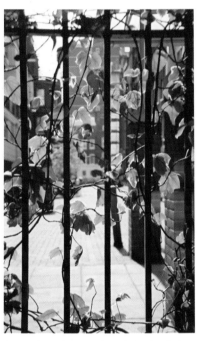

Secure boundary to a hospital school play area.

Notes

29 NHS Estates. **HTM 85: Fire precautions in existing hospitals.** HMSO, 1994, and HTM 86: Fire risk assessment in hospitals. HMSO, 1994.

of the furniture (chair sizes, table heights and numbers of computer workstations) will be significantly different for each age group. In some cases, classrooms may be combined in an open plan facility (see Case Study 2), whereas in others they are better kept as separate rooms.

Generally, a hospital education facility will need one or more classroom spaces for six to eight pupils and smaller satellite teaching spaces which benefit from quiet and separation. There may be a need for occasional access to a larger space (which could be created by combining two smaller spaces) for events, workshops etc. A school serving a psychiatric unit may require a wider range of spaces for specialist rooms (for example for design and technology, see Section A7.6 and B8).

"The space of the secondary school resource base needs to be highly adaptable for different classes. For example, we may need to set up a sewing machine for a design and technology class." Secondary level teacher and assistant head of education in a hospital school.

Diagram illustrating the multiple range of activities that are likely to take place in a classroom, and the need for flexibility. In the first case a range of activities involving three different Key Stage groups are happening simultaneously, whereas in the second case the space has been cleared for a single Key Stage 2 group P.E. lesson. The necessity for a dedicated store area is clearly illustrated.

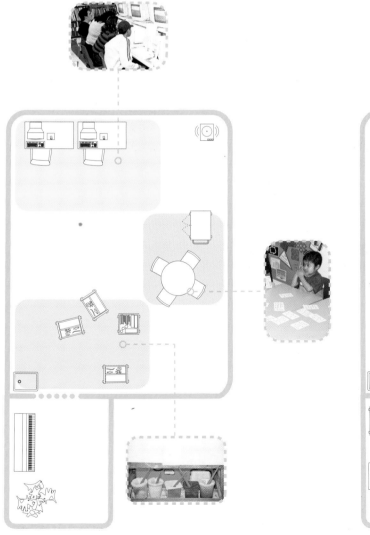

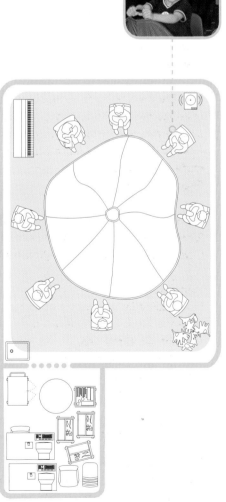

Key Stage 1
Key Stage 2
Key Stage 3

Following analysis of case study examples, and the experience of observing teaching groups in action, it is suggested that an area of between 5m^2 and 9m^2 per pupil place is allowed for class-rooms, (a satellite teaching space may need less area per pupil unless the space is for practical activities or it is used by pupils who need a large amount of medical equipment). The range relates primarily to the amount of equipment that the pupil profile tends to have (see Section A7). For example, an educational facility providing mostly for wheelchair and bedbound (but able to come to the classroom) pupils or pupils with drips should calculate at the high end of the range. A facility catering mostly for mobile pupils with no equipment should calculate at the low end. Facilities catering for pupils with mental health problems, however, should calculate the area at the high end of the range, since many pupils with mental disorders learn better in a spacious environment. Flexibility of arrangement and use are key issues to be borne in mind at every stage in the development of the design. Wheelchair users should be able to freely navigate in a classroom without feeling that they are inconveniencing others.

B2.1   Classroom

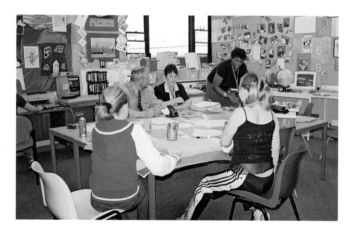

Key Stage 3 pupils at work in a classroom.

A hospital schoolroom is similar to a mainstream primary schoolroom in that it is multi-purpose and accommodates a wide range of activities including practical and art work. But it will tend to be used by a cross section of age groups, sometimes the full range of school-age pupils.

A consequence of mixed age groups means that teachers are less likely to address the class as a whole. A more likely pattern is groups of different levels at different tables or individuals working alone at tables or with computers. Flexibility is the key to classroom layouts, particularly where a space accommodates primary and secondary levels in a single teaching session.

The size of a classroom will vary depending on the nature of the facility and the pupil profile. Decisions about the appropriate area allowance should be based on a detailed analysis of the patient profile.

From studies of current practice, the optimum class size appears to be around six to eight pupils. This is based on a suggested maximum teaching ratio of 1:6. Classrooms which are too small to comfortably sit a group of six to eight create serious problems for teachers and pupils (concentration, health and safety (tripping over drip leads) etc.).

The under-provision of area for classrooms at the planning stage of a hospital project is the single most significant factor in reducing the effectiveness of the education facility.

A number of classroom arrangements observed in hospital schools.

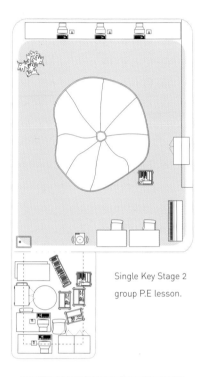

Single Key Stage 2 group P.E lesson.

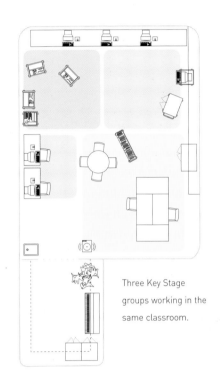

Three Key Stage groups working in the same classroom.

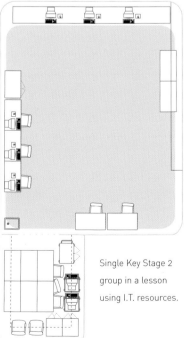

Single Key Stage 2 group in a lesson using I.T. resources.

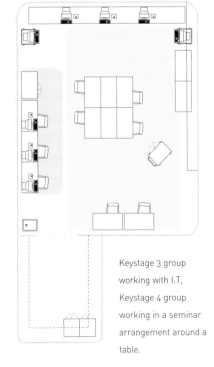

Keystage 3 group working with I.T, Keystage 4 group working in a seminar arrangement around a table.

Key Stage 1
Key Stage 2
Key Stage 3
Key Stage 4

B2.2   Satellite spaces

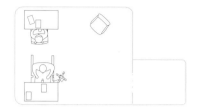 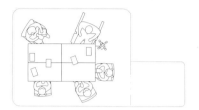 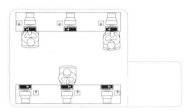

Some uses of satellite teaching spaces.

Satellite teaching spaces are important for providing quieter study areas (particularly for older pupils who may need to focus on quieter study activities, for one-to-one teaching, music lessons, or pupils who may need to withdraw from the main classroom).

Satellite teaching spaces may be used for holding public examinations, when necessary. Alternatively, in smaller facilities, a non-teaching space, such as a staff room or the head teacher's office, may be used for this purpose. The main characteristics of the examination space are that it should be quiet, well lit, secure and free from possible interruption. It should also simulate the conditions of a mainstream school examination room.

B2.3   Ward teaching

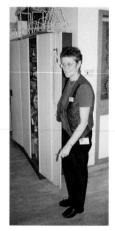 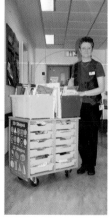 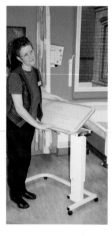

Ward teaching: Lockable storage cupboard; ward teaching trolley; adjustable height and angle table for bedside use.

"In a single teaching session I might see a new pupil with their leg sticking out in a plaster cast, in hospital for just the morning, a pupil who is in for several months for an intensive chemotherapy treatment, and one who comes in weekly for dialysis, who I have been teaching for five years. I will need to ensure that on my trolley I have enough material for all of them, (and for the pupil who was unexpectedly discharged and went home)." Ward Teacher in a hospital school.

Current NHS Estates guidance on ward design should be taken into account when considering provision for ward teaching[30]. Pupils who are not well enough to come to the school are taught on the wards (usually, but not always, 1:1). Examples of specialist wards where children are taught at the bedside are renal, oncology and those dedicated to the treatment of cystic fibrosis.

Notes

30 See NHS Estates. HBN 04: **Inpatient accommodation – options for choice.** HMSO, 1997.

Ward teachers often use a trolley which holds a basic set of materials topped up daily. The design of the trolley (see Section B6.8) is important, since this will carry key teaching resources.

The trolleys are usually stored centrally. Local ward storage of some materials is very important (see Section B3.1.1). Ward teaching is resource intensive: teachers usually set up work for a number of pupils and then spend a period of time with each pupil in turn.

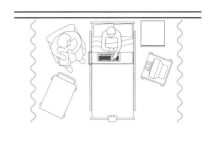

Diagram illustrating the constraints of space in a ward teaching situation.

B2.4 Isolation teaching

For pupils with a vulnerable immune system, visitors, including teachers, have to pass through a lobby to the bedroom. Equipment has to be cleaned or in some cases new (to prevent risk of infection from previous users) and delivered in sealed packs. In other cases, materials may have to be destroyed after use or thoroughly disinfected. The teacher will need access to a washing/disinfecting facility and a photocopier since some teaching materials will need to be disposable to prevent contamination (see Section A7.5). Storage for duplicate educational resources close to the location of the isolation teaching is advisable.

B2.5 Facilities without dedicated classrooms

In some cases, permanent teacher provision at the hospital may not be warranted (for example, in a small local facility where the frequency of school-age admissions is low). In such cases, teaching will be provided by the LEA on demand. The following equipment should be provided for these situations:

- Access to a phone, fax machine and email for the teachers. This is essential to allow the teachers fast access to the home school.
- A lockable cupboard for teaching materials. This should be approximately 2m high, 450mm deep and 1200mm wide. If the facility requires the teacher to travel between floors or long distances from the storage cupboard, a trolley will need to be provided and housed. The approximate dimensions for a ward teaching trolley are 700mm high, 500mm wide and 700mm long (not including the handle).
- Provision of a bedside computer is particularly important in these situations, since it allows fast access to a wide range of teaching and learning resources. Facilities that do not have a dedicated classroom with ICT resources should ensure the provision of Internet and audio-visual resources at the bedside. These should be permanent, so that the pupil can continue to have access to learning materials when the teacher is absent.

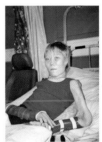

"It is hard to study on the ward as people have television on. I have used computers a lot, as I broke both arms and couldn't write well, but I could still type. Ideally there would be more laptops available for people working in bed, and internet access too." Pupil aged 18 years in a hospital school.

Where pupils in hospital are able to go to a schoolroom, the level of concentration is higher and the effectiveness of education delivery is far greater. Therefore, this should always be the option of choice wherever possible. Learning is also a social activity.

B3   Non-teaching areas

B3.1   Storage

In the Case Studies made for this guidance, storage was ranked second in importance (after classroom size) of priority requirements for a hospital education facility.

B3.1.1 Teaching storage

There are three key locations for teaching storage:
- a central storeroom;
- classroom storeroom;
- ward storage.

A centralised storeroom is essential for assisting in teaching efficiency. It is needed for shared equipment such as laptops and duplicate resources used in isolation rooms and on wards. Such a store may need to be large enough to house computer trolleys and, in some cases, occasional furniture. The area of the central storeroom will vary according to the individual facility need; for example, in situations where there are many teachers engaged in ward teaching, more central storage will be needed for materials and trolleys (see section B2.5).

Classrooms should have a dedicated storage room opening directly to the teaching space. In a single classroom, different pupils might be using various resources (for example, some may be painting and some running a modern languages CD-ROM); the teacher must have direct access to the resources required. An area of around 1m² to 1.4m² per pupil space for classroom storage is recommended (in addition to the area allocation for teaching space per pupil). Teachers should not have to leave the classroom to retrieve materials.

Transporting teaching materials between areas wastes time and in some cases is inappropriate because of the risks of cross infection (see Section B2.4). Lockable storage on the wards is therefore

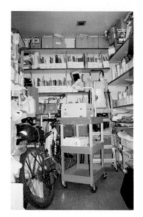

Classroom storeroom.

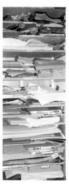

Art materials storage.

Useful storeroom layouts. Information taken from: "Art Accommodation in Secondary Schools", Building Bulletin 89, Figure 2/10 p 22.

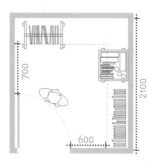
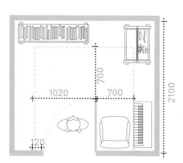
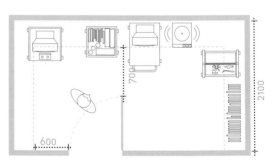

essential (at least a lockable cupboard large enough to store computer equipment, art material and a range of books and CD-ROMs). The minimum recommendation is for a lockable cupboard approximately 2m high, 450mm deep and 1200mm wide.

B3.1.2 Administration storage

Teachers update teaching record sheets for each patient daily (see Section A3). This generates a great deal of hard copy records that need to be stored. It is inevitable that as data storage becomes more electronically based, there will be less pressure for on-site hard copy storage. However, adequate provision will need to be made for hard copy storage of pupil records which is likely to be required in the immediate future.

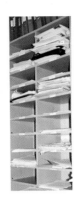

B3.1.3 Personal storage

There should be lockable storage space for all staff. This might be provided as full length lockers for the personal effects of each member of staff, or hooks and shelves in a lockable staff room.

B3.2 Entrance areas

If the hospital education facility is located in one main group of spaces, it should have an entrance or threshold area. These areas can serve a number of useful functions. They will announce the presence of the facility to hospital staff and parents. They should provide a security checkpoint (either as a surveyed reception area, lock system or both). They can also usefully showcase the pupils' work and provide a helpful psychological boundary between medical and educational worlds.

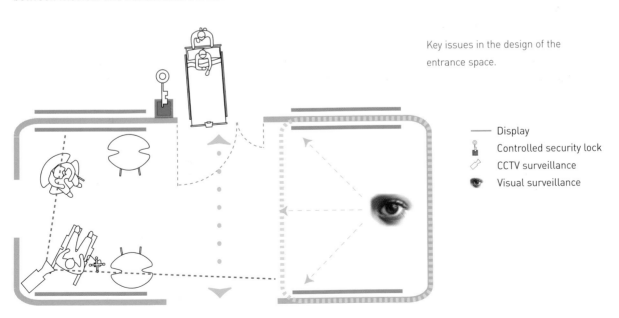

Key issues in the design of the entrance space.

—— Display
Controlled security lock
CCTV surveillance
Visual surveillance

The entrance should be spacious enough to allow access for beds and wheelchairs[31]. The entrance space may be economically made by linking the circulation area to an appropriate administration space.

Sometimes, where for example the hospital education facility is small or fully integrated with a single ward, the entrance and arrival point might be shared with the ward reception. Entrance spaces should be welcoming and help visitors with orientation.

B3.3   Administration office(s)

The minimum requirement for any school with full time teaching provision is an administrative office providing a base for staff. In a suite of spaces, this should be located near to the entrance of the facility. It should be equipped with a telephone, fax machine and one computer workstation per staff member.

If there is a head teacher, he/she needs a separate office for dealing with administration and management issues, conducting meetings with parents, pupils and medical staff, and storing secure records.

B3.4   Staff room

A staff room is essential. It should be large enough for work preparation, which will require desks and computer provision, and for social use, such as breaks and meals. It should provide a pleasant and restful environment. The staff room should be suf-ficiently large to allow for general meetings. This room may also be used for occasional quiet teaching activities such as educational examinations. In some situations the staff room is used as a resource store or base, but this is not recommended, since it reduces the area for key staff activities. The staff room should have a telephone, fax machine and photocopier and may need to accommodate records. There should be tea-making facil-ities, a microwave oven and an area for notices. The hospital's policy on smoking would need to be adhered to.

B3.5   Ancillary spaces

Some spaces might be provided within or shared with the health trust provision, depending on the needs and size of the particular hospital education facility. These spaces are referred to in this guidance as 'ancillary', since they have a relationship to educa-tional activities.

Linking ancillary spaces with the hospital education facility can be extremely useful, particularly for young people, where there may be a more extended time period of use. Examples of such spaces are kitchens, gyms (which may be part of the youth

Notes

31 For further information on designing for accessibility, contact the Centre for Accessible Environments
http://www.cae.org

worker's or physiotherapist's domain) or rooms used for social activities. The wider context in which the hospital education facility is placed must therefore be taken into account, particularly the spaces adjoining the education facility, to ensure the maximum benefit from the siting of the facility.

Kitchens may be regarded as either a teaching or ancillary space depending on their use. Some kitchens are used as teaching rooms (for example, in food technology classes) and others are a place for staff to make drinks. Current hospital education facilities which have a kitchen area suitable for teaching regard this as a very positive resource for both food technology and life skills. Food technology areas should have an allowance of around 6m^2 per pupil, assuming that group sizes would be relatively small. Wheelchair users will require more space, around 9m^2 per pupil[32].

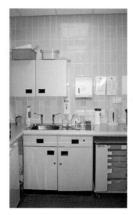

Kitchen used for teaching in a hospital school.

B3.6 Toilets

The teaching facility should have toilets for pupils although some pupils may need to return to the ward to use the toilet for treatment monitoring (for example, sample taking).

At least one toilet for each sex in the facility should be wheelchair-accessible[33]. Toilets should be easily and quickly accessible from all teaching spaces and large enough to allow for the changing of clothes (pupils may need to be assisted by a member of staff). Reference should be made to relevant NHS Estates guidance[34].

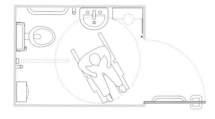

Wheelchair W.C. layout. Refer to: **Access for Disabled People to School Buildings**, Building Bulletin 91, p 32 and current NHS guidance.

Door locks should have an override so that they can be opened from the outside. Toilets should be equipped with a panic button or pull cord (pull cords should not be used in mental health provision). Some basins should be at a low height for wheelchair users and small children. Mirrors may cause distress to patients undergoing certain treatments. The patient profile of the facility should be considered before deciding to include mirrors. Roller-towel machines should not be used for reasons of patient safety. Storage for sterile sample equipment may be required in or near the education facility toilets. (A small, wall-mounted, lockable cupboard is sufficient.)

Separate staff toilets must also be provided. Staff should also have access to a shower, which may be shared by other hospital staff and be part of the general trust provision.

Notes

32 A proposal to include kitchens as part of the hospital education provision should be discussed with the health and safety representative.

33 See Department for Education and Employment. **Building Bulletin 91: Access for disabled people to school buildings - management and design guide**. TSO, 1999.

34 See NHS Estates. **HBN 40: Common activity spaces, Vol. 2 – Treatment areas**, HMSO, 1995 (this guidance is currently under review).

B3.7   Circulation

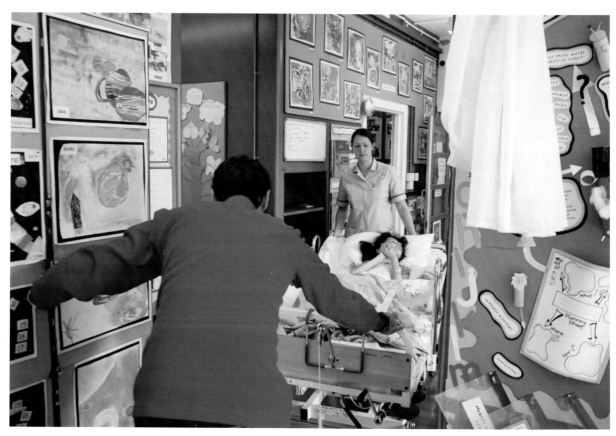

Pupil in a bed arriving at the classroom.

Since teaching spaces will need to accommodate pupils in beds and wheelchairs (from which limbs in plaster casts may protrude), it is important to ensure that access along corridors and into rooms is easy and unimpeded. NHS Estates' Health Building Note 40 gives extensive information on the parameters for various corridor and door arrangements[35]. Corridors of around 2000mm width allow for beds and wheelchairs to circulate with room for others to pass safely. Circulation and other areas must comply with the requirements of relevant fire safety standards[36].

B4   Outside space

Case study examples which had dedicated outside space were frequently used and popular with staff and pupils. PE, games, social events, fundraising activities, drama and music performance are examples of the multiple activities that outside spaces play host to. All new education facilities should have an outside school area.

Younger children might be more interested in the play aspect of the outside space, but for older children and young people the provision of a more reflective place (possibly a landscaped or planted area) can be very beneficial.

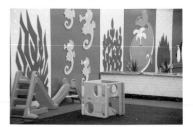

Roof converted to make outdoor play space.

Notes

35 See NHS Estates. **HBN 40: Common activity spaces, Vol. 4 - Circulation areas.** HMSO, 1995 (this guidance is currently under review).

36 For example, see NHS Estates. **HTM 85: Fire precautions in existing hospitals.** HMSO, 1994, and **HTM 86: Fire risk assessment in hospitals.** HMSO, 1994.

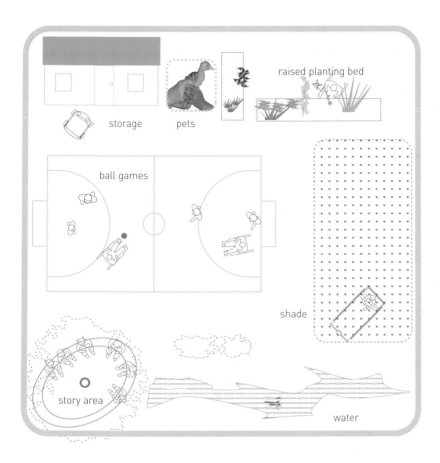

storage

pets

raised planting bed

ball games

shade

story area

water

Range of possible activities for an outside space (not to scale).

As in the design of interior spaces, it is important to ensure that there is plenty of scope for flexibility in the way the outdoor space can be used. Design teams need to check whether the various activities that might take place (storytelling, games of softball, summer parties) can all be accommodated at different times in the space. Popular games such as softball are informal; thus, standard court dimensions do not need to be applied.

"If I could change anything about the school I would have another place to go to for breaks and lunch time." Primary age pupil.

B4.1   Location

External areas should be at the same level as the main teaching spaces, directly and horizontally accessible, without the need for lifts or ramps. Rooftops provide a good opportunity for a play space if imaginatively designed and easily accessible for wheelchairs and beds.

Direct access and good visibility from the classroom is recommended, allowing the space, particularly at primary level, to be used as an extension of the classroom.

Attention should be paid to the needs of adjacent spaces when siting outside play areas. For example, noise generated in the play area could be unwelcome to adjacent ward areas. Equally, the educational facility should not be overlooked by non-related areas, such as an adult ward.

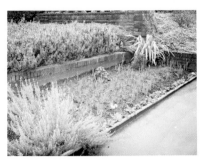

Garden planted with spring bulbs by hospital school pupils.

B4.2   Landscaping

A creatively planted garden can be a very welcome place for pupils and staff. Although gardening may not be an appropriate activity for some pupils for health and safety reasons, it will be a welcome activity for others. The degree to which successful gardening is possible will depend on the siting and orientation of the play area.

For wheelchair users, a raised planting bed is preferable. The planting and ongoing maintenance of a garden area should be discussed: whether it will be the responsibility of the hospital or school. The therapeutic and contemplative qualities of water are well known. However, if a pond or water feature is considered in the design, pupil safety is of primary importance.

Well drained, impact absorbing play surfaces are acceptable and allow year round use[37]. If the area is suitable (that is, large enough and with good orientation for sunlight and growth), a lawn area is popular as a play surface.

B4.3   Equipment

Seating and a table should be provided (these may need to be kept in a storage shed when not in use). There is a range of outdoor play equipment available for all age groups, and it is important to look at how these might overlap and coexist in the layout of a play space at the planning stage.

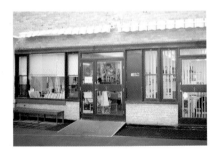

Retractable canopy to provide shade to outside area.

Moveable play equipment has the advantage that it can be rearranged. If the space is large, fixed play equipment can be considered, either purpose designed or proprietary[38].

B4.4   Shade

Shaded areas should be provided in external spaces. This can be achieved either by erecting fixed structures (for example, lattices and pergolas) and planting suitable plants/shrubs or by moveable devices such as operable canopies. Some pupils, for example those undergoing chemotherapy, should not be exposed to direct sunlight, but will want to be able to go outside in a protected (shady) environment. A covered external area has the double benefit of providing shade and allowing the outside area to be used even in bad weather.

Notes

37 Useful guidance on the range of suitable products is available from the National Playing Fields Association **http://www.npfa.co.uk**

38 See Department for Education and Employment. **Building Bulletin 71. The outdoor classroom: educational use, landscape design and management of school grounds.** TSO, 1999, for information on outdoor space design for mainstream schools.

B4.5   Outdoor storage

A lockable storage shed that can adequately contain large toys (such as tricycles) and play equipment should be included.

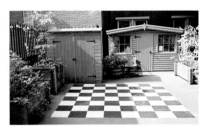

Storage for play equipment in an outside area.

B4.6   Outdoor security and safety

The outdoor play space should be for school use only and access to and from the play area should be strictly controllable from the school area alone.

As ball games are likely to be played, thought should be given to a means of enclosing the area. Full netting (such as tennis-court netting) to the sides and over the top is effective, although not visually pleasing. For security fencing, 2.4m is regarded as an adequate height, but 3m is a more effective height to contain stray balls. For rooftop areas, 4m is preferable.

B5   Design of elements

B5.1   Materials and surfaces

For teaching and medical staff, the wards and education areas are their permanent place of work; for the pupils they are, temporarily, their whole environment.

The design of surfaces in the educational facility should therefore be to a high aesthetic standard, and all surfaces chosen to enhance the coherence and overall delight of the spaces. A full range of material and surface choices, within obvious practical limits, should be considered.

It is important to discuss the cleaning regime as part of the design process, since this will affect the selection of the surfaces and coatings. The variation in patient profile between different education facilities will be reflected in different requirements. The specification of all surfaces should also comply with current Firecode guidance[39].

If specific art or installation work is being considered (including special wall and floor treatments), this should be incorporated into the design from the earliest stage. Pupils' work will form a major part of the display in classrooms, and the design should enable this both visually and practically.

Hospital classrooms should look and feel like mainstream classrooms as much as possible. Inevitably, sick children will occasionally be ill during teaching sessions. Easy to clean and hygienic surfaces are recommended where this is likely[40].

Notes

39 See NHS Estates. **HTM 85: Fire precautions in existing hospitals.** HMSO, 1994 and **HTM 86: Fire risk assessment in hospitals.** HMSO, 1994.

40 Refer to NHS Estates. **HFN 30: Infection control in the built environment.** TSO, 2002.

B5.2   Floors

The range of floor finishes which are suitable will vary depending on the patient profile of the education facility. For example, in an education facility attached to a mental health unit, a complete range of finishes including wood strip, wood block, carpet and vinyl floor finishes may be suitable. For units which cater for patients with mental health problems only, the infection control measures will not be as stringent as those required in a school which deals with a range of medical conditions. In areas for gym or assembly, a harder surface (wood or vinyl) may be most suitable, whereas in a classroom, the acoustic properties of carpets might be preferable. In toilets, vinyl flooring is the most appropriate specification. In hospital education facilities where infection control is vital, the specification of floor finish will be more limited and will need to comply with specific NHS Estates guidance[41]. For example, while carpets are considered to give a friendlier feel to the space and can have acoustic benefits, they are not always ideal for infection control reasons. The use of carpeting in certain areas should therefore be discussed with all interested parties at the planning stage.

Materials and surface coatings in certain circumstances can be pollutants or be toxic. This applies particularly to synthetic resins, which may be especially harmful to patients with respiratory conditions[42].

B5.3   Walls

Appropriate wall surfaces include safety glass, laminates, wood panelling or board, textiles[43] and plastered finishes. The precise selection and composition will depend on the patient profile and other requirements of the particular education facility. However, where transparency is desirable (for example, to common spaces) safety glass may be appropriate. This should be framed to look like a window to avoid safety hazards for the visually impaired.

For areas where pinboards will be fixed for the display of work, plastered walls provide a good, flat substrate surface. In toilets, plastered walls allowing paint finishes are recommended. In wet areas (washrooms with showers, areas around sinks) ceramic tiles are suitable. Different surfaces can be used to help define areas (for example, textiles might be considered for quieter areas for storytelling)[44].

B5.4   Ceilings

Ceilings are sometimes referred to as the forgotten sixth plane of a room. The ceiling, as a surface, should be carefully considered. Any servicing tasks accommodated within the ceiling should be framed within an overall design idea which is appropriate to, and

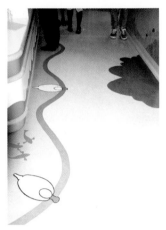

Patterning to floor in a children's ward.

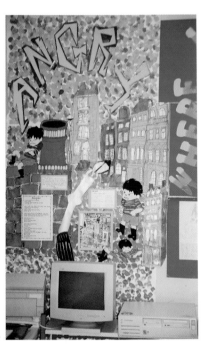

Wall display.

Notes

41 See NHS Estates. **HBN 23: Hospital accommodation for children and young people**. TSO, 2003 (forthcoming), and NHS Estates. **HFN 30: Infection control in the built environment**. TSO, 2002.

42 See Bjorn Berge. **The ecology of building materials**, Architectural Press, 2001.

43 For all textile specifications, infection control must be borne in mind: refer to NHS Estates. **HFN 30: Infection control in the built environment**. TSO, 2002.

44 In all situations textiles should conform to the guidance on infection control, see NHS Estates. **HFN 30: Infection control in the built environment**. TSO, 2002.

in tune with, the feel and scale of the room. Easy access to services must be provided for maintenance.

The ceiling can also provide sound absorption which is useful where a variety of activities may take place simultaneously.

Ceilings are commonly used for fixing artwork such as mobiles, and they should be robust enough to allow for this without sustaining damage.

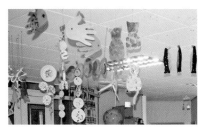

Ceiling display.

B5.5 Doors and windows

Vision panel heights: Information taken from: **Access for Disabled People to School Buildings**, Building Bulletin 91, p.29.

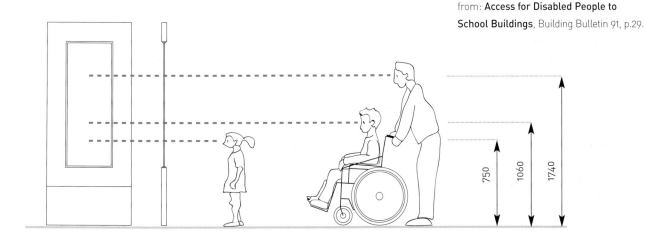

750 1060 1740

Doors should be wide enough to allow wheelchairs and beds to pass through comfortably and safely (see Section A7.4). A common arrangement is to have a pair of doors of unequal leaf size with an overall width of 1300mm (split into 900mm and 400mm leaves) which allows a bed or wheelchair to pass. If doors are set close to a corner of a corridor, they may need to be significantly wider to accommodate the turning geometry of beds. If it works with the room layout, a single door of 1300mm, which allows easy passage with no extra effort, is the optimum solution.

Design teams should ensure that any special equipment that is likely to be used by a pupil attending the education facility can be accommodated by the specified door width. Allowance should be made for lower height vision panels for small children and those in wheelchairs for both internal and external doors.

Windows should be designed to prevent anyone from getting out or in for reasons of pupil security (100mm maximum opening).

Some pupils may be at risk of self-harm. All glazing should be safety glass. Window heights from the floor should allow a reasonable view for a wheelchair user (the eye-level zone of children in wheelchairs varies from 900mm to 1150mm). Window controls (ironmongery, blinds) should be set at a maximum height of 1200mm to allow access.

Windows should not create a hazard, either inside or outside, when opened.

B5.6   Colour and texture

Selecting good colour schemes is important. The colour scheme for the project should be considered as a whole so that different spaces and colours work in a complementary manner. Careful use of colour can relieve monotony and contribute very positively to the experience of the environment[45].

Calm, relatively neutral surface colours are preferable in a teaching space that will tend to be animated by pupils' colourful displays.

Lighting colour temperature will have a marked effect on the colour rendition of any finish, and the lamp type should be considered when selecting colours. A colour test might be appropriate. Colour and texture of all surfaces will have an effect on the amount of daylight reflection within a space. Light surface colours should be chosen, particularly where natural light is restricted.

Colour in design is part of the aesthetic intention of the whole, and the design life of the space should be taken into account when considering specific colour schemes. Some elements of the design (for example, wall colour) might be changed sooner than others (for example, tables and chairs, or floor finishes)[46].

B6   Furniture and fittings

Furniture and fittings chosen for a hospital school need to take the following factors into account:
- All ages may be taught in the same space.
- A wide range of practical and non-practical activities take place in the same room, often using the same furniture.
- Some pupils will be in wheelchairs or using various types of walking aid.

Design teams should aim to make flexible, open and light spaces with the minimum fixed furniture and the greatest opportunity for flexibility (see Section B2.1). It is recommended that standard proprietary suppliers are used for the basics (tables, chairs, plan chests etc.) since this enables replacements and additional orders to be made simply and quickly. BS 5873 is the key standard for educational furniture. A certain amount of customisation (colours, for example) can be used to make these items work with the design. Ensure that colour specification will permit reordering.

"Doors that you have to pull to open are a bit of a problem. I do have an auxiliary who opens doors for me, but I find this very intrusive, and would love to be able to go about school on my own like any other pupil. Pushing doors is no problem as my electric wheelchair is very strong and can give me the strength to do that." Member of Whizz Kidz Childrens and Young Persons Advisory Team. (Whizz Kidz is an organisation dedicated to improving the life of disabled children in the U.K.)

Notes

45 See Sarah Hosking and Liz Haggard. **Healing the hospital environment.** E & FN Spon, London, 1999, ISBN: 0419231706, pp. 117-123.

46 See Department for Education and Employment. **Furniture and equipment in schools: a purchasing guide.** Managing school facilities Guide 7. TSO, 2000, pp. 79-80.

Adjustable furniture is likely to be required, for example to assist wheelchair and bed bound pupils. For a full treatment of issues relating to the selection and specification of furniture and equipment, see Furniture and equipment in schools[47].

B6.1   Ergonomics

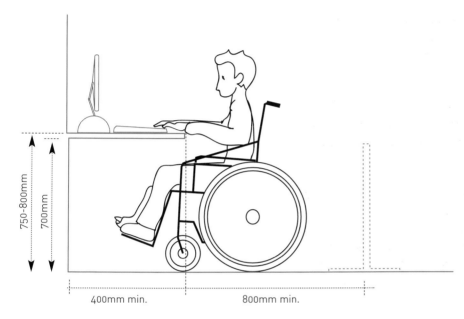

All pupils, whatever their age or disability, should be able to work as comfortably as possible in the classroom[48]. The design team should liaise closely with all interested parties to ensure that a reasonable provision for height, range and disability can be accommodated, reflecting the patient profile of the facility. For most pupils who use the schoolroom, standard table and chair heights will be suitable. The simplest approach is to provide a range of chair and table sizes to suit the appropriate age range with a few spare items kept in the classroom store.

Wheelchair users must be able to reach equipment (for example, keyboards). Some pupils will need to use a touch screen computer rather than a keyboard. In such cases, teachers will normally require an adjustable height trolley or table.

Adjustable height worktops are useful in a kitchen area. Access to sinks in classrooms for wheelchair users should be ensured. The needs of all users will need to be taken into account in the design and specification of sanitary fittings[49]. Grab handles and easy on/off taps will need to be considered.

Notes

47 Department for Education and Employment. **Furniture and equipment in schools: a purchasing guide**. Managing school facilities Guide 7. TSO, 2000.

48 See http://www.doh.gov.uk./dda/index.htm for further information on ergonomic issues.

49 See Department for Education and Employment. **Building Bulletin 91: Access for disabled people to school buildings - management and design guide**. TSO, 1999, and Department for Education and Skills. **Building Bulletin 77: Designing for pupils with special educational needs**. 1997, for useful information on hygiene for special needs pupils.

B6.2   Tables

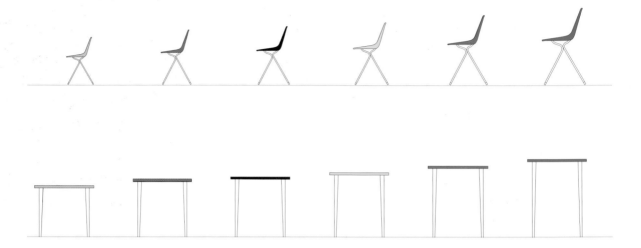

Range of furniture to BS 5873 sizemarks.
Refer to: **Furniture and equipment in Schools: A Purchasing guide** DfEE 2000.

Teachers need to be able to move tables easily to rearrange a space to suit changing activities. They may even want to store them away to create a clear space. Teachers generally prefer this option to folding tables which they regard as unnecessarily time consuming. As well as being easy to move, tables should be sturdy and practical. Standard school tables with tough laminated surfaces and firmly applied edgings are a practical and reliable choice.

Table heights need to conform to the pupil stature profile and to co-ordinate with chair heights. For bed-bound pupils, tables with pivoting tops are also recommended. Refer to **Furniture and equipment in schools**[50] for more information on tables.

"I arrange the class to make one large table in the centre with a wide space for circulation around. I need to be able see every child. The space is regularly re-arranged for different activities. We move tables out into the corridor space for some individual teaching." Teacher in a hospital school.

B6.3   Benching/worktops

Fixed benching/worktops along the walls of at least part of a teaching space provide a useful worktop area for standing height working and display. Perimeter benching may also be used for desktop computers (although this can limit the flexibility of a layout, see Section B6.4).

A sink should be included in a run of benching in each of the main classrooms (see Section B7.4) but be far enough away from electrical equipment. Fixed benching must be at a suitable height to accommodate the likely pupil range[51]. Two runs of benching at different heights may be considered (where space allows) where the full age range is taught together. Fixed benching/worktops can usefully be combined with under-bench storage. This can reduce the space available for pupils to sit at the bench, although storage units on castors can be wheeled away to allow pupils to sit at the bench when necessary.

Notes

50 Department for Education and Employment. **Furniture and equipment in schools: a purchasing guide**. Managing school facilities Guide 7. TSO, 2000.

51 See **http://www.whizz-kidz.org.uk** for information on this and other issues related to wheelchair users.

B6.4   Work surfaces for ICT

Hospital pupils will use desktop computers and laptops. Desktop computers may be housed on a fixed surface such as a perimeter bench or on computer trolleys. The advantage of fixed workstations is that power and network cabling can be managed in a neat and controlled manner using service conduits[52].

Relevant sitting heights should be provided for pupils using computers. Computer trolleys allow teachers to arrange the space to suit a particular group. Since the make up of a group will vary from hour to hour, such flexibility is essential. Trolleys can be moved out of the classroom altogether to clear a space. It is important that the classroom storeroom is large enough to house several trolleys (see Section B6.8) because storing furniture in corridors may infringe fire and health and safety regulations.

Desktop computers on trolleys are also recommended for bedside teaching where some patients (for example, those with limited mobility) may need adapted keyboards or touch-screen interactivity. Computer equipment on the wards is particularly vulnerable to theft; thus, security measures, such as device locks, should be considered.

The size of the trolley is important given the limited space around the hospital bed. One of the hospital schools visited as part of this study designed a special 'slimline' computer trolley (550mm wide by 550mm deep) which takes up less space.

Trolleys should have brakes for safety. Those that have adjustable components (for example, to allow access to interactive screens) should ideally be adjustable while the equipment is mounted, avoiding the need to remove equipment before adjusting.

With the increasing use of wireless technology, cable management is likely to become less of an issue and lead to more flexible arrangements allowing pupils to use laptops on any suitable surface. Laptops can be easily managed at the bedside by many pupils and be stored on resource trolleys allowing them to be moved to where they are needed. Where they are run by battery, facilities for efficient recharging should be provided (see Section B7.2).

B6.5   Seating

Chair heights should co-ordinate with tables. Polypropylene chairs, which are stackable and easy to clean, are suitable for basic provision as they are often robust, relatively light and can easily be stacked up and stored when the space needs to be reconfigured.

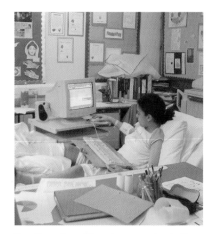

Year 8 pupil working at a computer in the education facility.

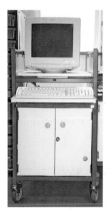

Slimline computer trolley designed by teaching staff for minimum space take-up in a ward teaching situation.

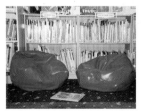

Seating for a quiet reading area.

Notes

52 See Department for Education and Employment. **Furniture and equipment in schools: a purchasing guide**. Managing school facilities Guide 7. TSO, 2000, pp. 51-2.

Other types of seating that may be considered include:
- stools to be used at standing height benching;
- adjustable office style chairs for use with computers;
- window seats with a view to a garden or play area (children, especially young children, like to perch in unconventional places);
- beanbags for soft informal areas.

B6.6   Display

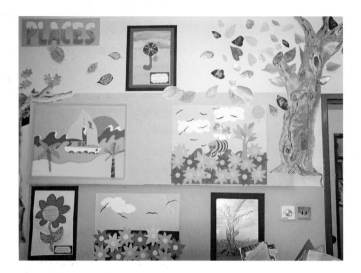

Display of pupils' work in an education facility.

It is important to allow space for two and three dimensional display of pupils' work and other inspirational materials. In the classroom this means providing a combination of flat wall surface and shelving.

Artwork in the corridors can signal the presence of the school to visitors, hospital staff and patients as well as enlivening the environment. Design for the display of artwork in corridors should be considered as part of the overall wall surface design. Where there are internal windows between corridors and class-rooms, display shelves can be incorporated into the design.

The requirements of Building Regulations and NHS Estates Firecode guidance should always be borne in mind where corridors are part of an escape route.

B6.7   Storage furniture

Shelves are useful in classrooms for exhibiting three dimensional displays and for local storage. But the main storage area should be a dedicated storeroom directly connected to the classroom (see Section B3.1.1). Adjustable shelves (moveable bracket systems are recommended) are preferable to take into account variations in the dimensions of stored materials and to provide flexibility.

Shelving provision should include storage for large objects (baskets for toys, flat paper storage etc.) and small objects such as arrays of CDs and books. For health and safety and convenience, teachers should not have to climb up to retrieve materials. This means that shelves above eye height (around 1500mm from the floor) are not recommended.

Wall cupboards are also commonly used. However, with a dedicated storeroom for each classroom, it should be possible to keep these to a minimum, since they reduce the area for display and can make the room feel cluttered.

Some floor mounted cupboards in the classroom should be provided for pupils so that they can access resources without having to go into the storeroom. Some of these cupboards should contain trays on runners so that resources can be easily seen, particularly if they are at low level and under fixed benching.

Trays can also be incorporated into trolleys (see Section B6.8) to allow resources to be easily transported across the hospital.

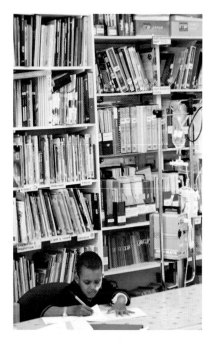

Library in a schoolroom.

B6.8 Trolleys

Bookshelf trolleys are common and useful in education facilities, since they allow materials to be taken on to the wards. Proprietary designs with moveable shelves and compartments which have been tested for stability are essential. The advantage of such moveable elements is that they allow a space to be relatively easily reconfigured for different teaching and learning situations in the classroom. Teaching resource trolleys are invaluable in hospital education, particularly for bedside teaching.

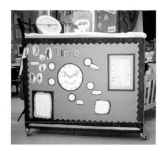

Bookshelf trolley.

Teachers need to take a variety of materials onto the ward including laptops, books, CDs, and art and craft materials. Storage for such trolleys must be taken into account at the planning stage. A trolley park or docking station at the school base associated with the central school storage is essential for facilities where there is extensive ward teaching.

Trolleys are also useful for transferring materials quickly to a satellite teaching room. Ward teaching trolleys should be robust in construction and have high quality braked castors or wheels so that they are easy to manoeuvre. They should have an adjustable handle height and a lockable section (for laptops and other valuables). Trays that allow resources to be transferred from units in the central storeroom or classroom are useful.

"I transport my teaching materials in a trolley, which I wheel around all day. This could be improved by adding lockable doors, as well as a few more drawers." Ward teacher.

A facility for recharging laptops and other equipment on the trolley is helpful. The approximate dimensions for a ward teaching trolley are 700mm high, 500mm wide and 700mm long (not including the handle).

B6.9   Partitioning

Teaching spaces may accommodate a number of different groups of pupils of different age bands; thus, flexibility of arrangement is particularly valuable where varying group numbers and activities have to be accommodated in a limited space. Moveable partitions or screens, which allow a space to be subdivided, should be considered. Dividing a teaching space can assist pupil concentration by providing visual and in some cases (depending on the type of screen) acoustic separation.

The three basic types of screen are described below.
- Curtains give visual separation. The fabric must have the appropriate fire retardance and resistance rating and comply with infection control guidance[53].
- Moveable screens (similar to those used in open plan offices) give limited acoustic separation. They have the advantage of mobility but space must be allowed for storing them when not in use.
- Acoustic screens provide acoustic separation and are most useful when there is an occasional need to open up two smaller spaces for activities such as music or drama in a bigger group. Such screens are expensive and can be cumbersome to operate. They will only give acoustic separation if they are fixed at the ceiling and floor and have a specifically designed heavy core.

Purpose designed units that combine storage or display with a screen may also be considered for visual separation.

Options for partitioning a classroom.

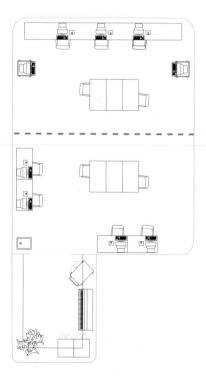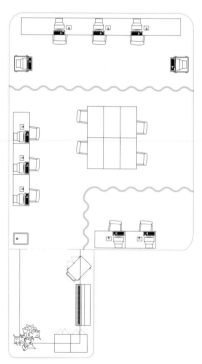

- - - - Acoustic screen

∼∼∼∼ Curtain partitioning/ moveable screens

Notes

53 See NHS Estates. **HFN 30: Infection control in the built environment.** TSO, 2002.

B7 Environmental design and services

B7.1 Lighting

In hospital school facilities, as in any educational accommodation, daylight should be the preferred form of lighting. Lighting design for schools (Building Bulletin 90[54]) gives useful guidance. Reference should also be made to standards for hospitals.

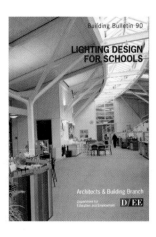

The figures for Standard Maintained Illuminance levels (in Lux) as suggested in Building Bulletin 90 are as follows:
- General teaching space: 300
- Teaching spaces with close and detailed work (for example, art and craft rooms):   500

Circulation spaces:
- Corridors and stairs: 80–120
- Waiting area: 175–250
- Reception area: 250–350

However, as hospital teaching rooms tend to be multi-purpose, it is advisable to design for the higher light level and provide flexible control. Dimmable lighting allows appropriate light levels to be set when using electronic whiteboards.

Although uniformity is desirable in some situations (for example, a teaching group working on a similar task), variation in natural and artificial lighting will help to create a varied and interesting world for the users of the facility.

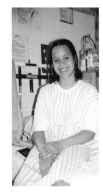

"I prefer to work in the schoolroom rather than in bed because it is quieter. The room is a bit dark. I would make it brighter and more colourful with posters and larger displays for art."
Year 7 pupil.

B7.1.1 Daylighting

The design for daylight should aim to keep the daylight level as even as possible throughout the space.

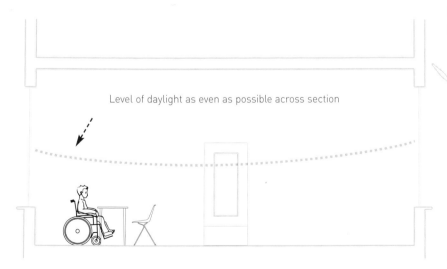

Level of daylight as even as possible across section

Notes

54 Department for Education and Employment. **Building Bulletin 90: Lighting design for schools.** TSO, 1999.

As in any classroom design, the best use of daylight should be made. Orientation will play an important part in deciding the best strategy. For example, south or west facing rooms will need to be equipped with blinds or shades to prevent glare, reflection and overheating problems resulting from too much direct sunlight. In single storey or upper floor locations, skylights are useful because of the high light to opening ratio that is achieved.

Some pupils, as a result of their particular conditions, should not be exposed to direct sunlight, and others might need to be protected from temperature fluctuations associated with direct sunlight.

7.1.2 Electric light

The electric lighting in a hospital education facility should complement daylighting, ensuring adequate lighting levels in all areas but also providing a comfortable and interesting lighting environment.

Uplighting may be considered for circulation areas and if chosen the ceiling colour should be pale (preferably white). Ceiling-mounted strip lighting should be avoided in circulation spaces: the rhythmic pattern created by a bed being wheeled along at regular speed can simulate stroboscopic lighting effects, which may cause some patients to suffer seizures.

In classrooms, fluorescent light fittings which combine some uplighting with downlighting are recommended, as they provide a good even spread of light and there is less contrast between the bright lights and unlit ceiling surfaces. Lamps with good colour-rendering properties should be chosen for teaching areas; this is particularly important for artwork.

Additional provision of special lights to enhance the dramatic feel of the space, or to vary lighting levels, is recommended. This can benefit musical and drama activities. Dimmable lighting is recommended in the classroom as it allows flexibility and mood shift. Dimming is also useful to ensure screens, monitors and whiteboards can be seen easily.

The design team should check that fluorescent units do not conflict with hearing-aid equipment[55]. The lighting scheme should include provision for emergency lighting in case of power failure or to aid means of escape in case of fire.

B7.1.3 Glare and reflection

It is important to design the layout of the space so that glare and reflection problems are avoided. This is particularly important for pupils with visual impairment. Examples of potential problems include:

Notes

55 The National Deaf Children Society (NDCS) state that "Fluorescent lighting is known to cause difficulties for some hearing-aid wearers, primarily when hearing aids are being used on the telecoil or "T" setting. Hearing-aid wearers are most likely to switch their hearing aid/s to the "T" setting in a room that is equipped with an induction loop system or when they are using certain assistive listening devices or a telephone with an inductive coupler. The design team should give consideration to the planned usage of the room and take this into account in the choice of appropriate lighting." See also NDCS/South West London NHS Trust/St George's Mental Health Trust. **Deaf children and young people in hospital**. 2000.

- a computer monitor placed in front of a window, where the level of brightness from the window is much greater than the screen brightness;
- pupils seeing a teacher in silhouette against a window or skylight[56];
- light from a window or a luminaire reflecting on a computer screen or a whiteboard.

Glare and reflection can be controlled by operable blinds, which are effective for dealing with light variations across the day. They are simple to use and provide an immediate and adaptable solution (see Section B7.1.3). Luminaires should be designed to minimise glare and reflections on both horizontal and vertical planes.

B7.1.4 Shading

Shading devices may be needed to reduce skylight, window glare or heat gain from direct sunlight. Fixed external shading (south and west elevations) is generally the most effective solution but internal blinds may be chosen for reasons of maintenance and cost. Internal blinds are very good for local adjustment, for example allowing pupils with visual impairment to optimise the lighting conditions for their work. Where infection control is required, internal blinds made of fabric should be avoided. Interstitial blinds (set between layers of double- or triple-glazed windows) have the advantage of being neatly contained and therefore do not collect dirt. This is the preferred arrangement in a hospital setting.

External and internal shading options should allow users easy control of the light condition.

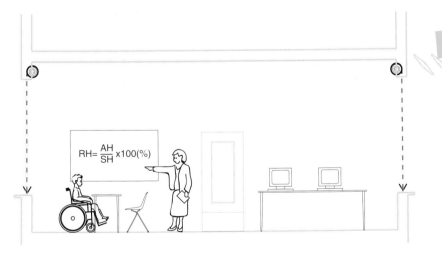

$$RH = \frac{AH}{SH} \times 100 (\%)$$

Notes

56 See Department for Education and Employment. **Building Bulletin 90: Lighting design for schools**. TSO, 1999, for a detailed exploration of window placement for classrooms.

B7.1.5 Visual impairment

A range of levels of visual difficulty[57] will be encountered in a hospital classroom, but some useful points to bear in mind are:

- Adjustable/dimmable task lighting is useful for carrying out specific work, such as looking at reflective screens.
- Routes within and to classrooms must be uncluttered (this is also important for ensuring fire escape routes are kept clear).
- Computers should be placed at 90° to windows to avoid glare and reflection on the screen.
- Adjustable blinds help control daylight and sunlight.
- Colour[58] and contrast can help visually-impaired pupils to navigate and establish orientation. Contrast colouring significant elements such as door handles, changes in direction in corridors and changes in floor levels, steps and skirting boards can give useful markers.

B7.2   Power supply

When planning the power supply to an education facility, the following specific considerations should be borne in mind:

- A pupil with a drip and pump might require up to three dedicated electrical sockets.
- With the requirement for flexible positioning of computer stations, printers, televisions and video players, teaching spaces should be supplied with sufficient socket outlets to allow all appliances likely to be used simultaneously to be individually supplied.
- Using a trunking system for supply is recommended, since it will allow flexibility in the placing and moving of socket positions, as long as sufficient outlets have been designed in to the supply.
- Pull-down, ceiling-mounted sockets give more flexibility for pupils with equipment to sit in the centre of the space.
- Teachers often prefer to equip bed-bound pupils with a battery-powered laptop computer for ergonomic and safety reasons. There should be a facility for recharging laptops and other battery-operated equipment when not in use, which could be an array of sockets located conveniently in a central resource store or classroom.
- Cabling to all classroom and bedside locations should allow for flexibility and changes in technology, particularly for ICT, and trunking which allows adaptation is essential. The increasing use of wireless and satellite technologies is likely to reduce cabling management and design issues.

B7.3   Educational technology

It should be possible to connect all computers to internal networks (allowing access to printers, scanners and other peripherals) and storage systems (including servers) to ensure

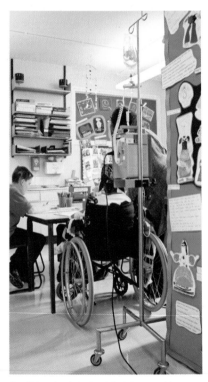

Pupil in wheelchair with drip stand in education facility.

Notes

57 See Department for Education and Employment. **Building Bulletin 94: Inclusive school design.** TSO, 2001.

58 ICI. **A design guide for the use of colour and contrast to improve the built environment for visually impaired people** 1997. CD-ROM and book. Available from Dulux Technical Advice Group. Tel: 0870 877 632.

that work can be stored in a safe and organised fashion. Fast and efficient access to the Internet should be planned in for all situations, whether in the classroom, in social spaces or at the bedside.

Networking and Internet access require careful planning and liaison with the hospital management body to ensure compatibility and service consistency. Bedside entertainment must complement and not intrude on the school's facilities and timetable. Space should be allowed for storing special needs ICT equipment such as alternative keyboards, joysticks, adjustable computer and mounting arms, and touch screens. ICT equipment storage should be secure.

"Ideally every bed head would be connected to the school server so that children can access educational or recreational resources from their beds in the middle of the night if they want to, if, for example, they are feeling pain and need a distraction." ICT Director and teacher in a hospital school.

B7.4 Water

All teaching spaces should be supplied with hot and cold water. For spaces where art is likely to take place (in most cases, this will be all classrooms), suitable sinks with drainers (for example, the Belfast type) should be provided. Smaller pupils will need to access the sink; thus designers should ascertain a good lower sink height which will suit the pupil profile. Taps should be of a lever design to assist special needs pupils who have difficulty with manipulation. Drinking water (normally provided throughout hospitals) should be available in all teaching areas.

B7.5 Ventilation and heating

Hospitals maintain high ambient temperatures. Set point temperatures will tend to be designed for bed bound patients. Teachers, parents and some pupils might find these temperatures too high in the school area. In particular, if games and activities are being undertaken, pupils can become hot quickly.

A teaching space will be accommodating pupils with a range of different thermal comfort requirements. Teachers in hospital education are adept at gauging the requirements of particular pupils and making adjustments to suit. It is vital that the educational areas have clear environmental controls, which provide fast and effective response so that teaching staff can modify the local environment in each room to suit the activities and pupils. It is important to ensure that users can easily understand how to make adjustments.

There are some situations where an air conditioning system might be necessary. For example, in inner city locations where air drawn directly from outside is polluted (and opening windows let in noise) or where there is a cooling requirement. Air-conditioning may also be necessary because of the medical condition of some pupils, for example those suffering from severe anaemia when dehydration is a danger and the humidity of

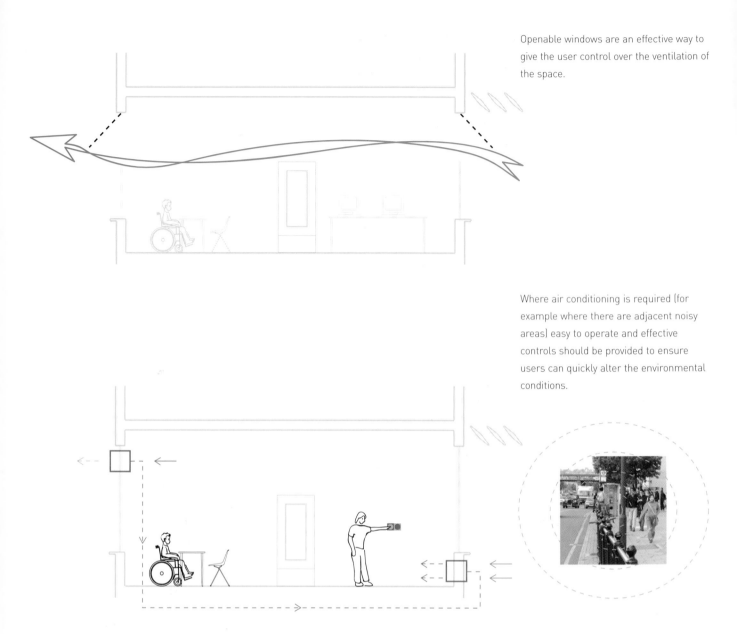

Openable windows are an effective way to give the user control over the ventilation of the space.

Where air conditioning is required (for example where there are adjacent noisy areas) easy to operate and effective controls should be provided to ensure users can quickly alter the environmental conditions.

the air may need to be controlled. The design of the building envelope should ensure that major heat losses or gains through the fabric do not distort the desired internal temperature.

Openable windows are desirable for all teaching and office areas (subject to the problem of noise and pollution mentioned above).

B7.6   Acoustics

The aim of good acoustic design is to enable people to hear clearly without distraction. Acoustic parameters used for mainstream schools may not necessarily be applicable to hospital facilities. In particular, group sizes are normally smaller and a teacher is rarely positioned at the front of the room, addressing the group. The room acoustics should be designed to suit the needs of individuals and small groups working alongside each other. The relatively reflective surfaces of some mainstream classrooms, designed to convey the voice of the teacher to all areas of the classroom as evenly as possible, are not generally suitable for a hospital education facility.

Moveable partitions might have sound absorbing material attached[59] to give some flexibility in the acoustic performance of the space. The ability to vary room acoustics might be useful in spaces used for a variety of group activities, including music (see Section A9.1).

Design teams should take account of pupils with hearing difficulties[60]. The range of hearing impairment will vary[61], but to ensure that children can make maximum use of their residual hearing, it is essential to be aware of their ability to hear sounds of different frequencies. It is helpful to consider the following:

- Noise levels: avoid conflicting and multiple sources of sound (and where this is impossible, for example in a classroom with multiple activities, consider some partitioning).
- Reverberation time and acoustic absorption need to be optimised for a teaching situation.
- Sound insulation of walls, floors and ceilings may be required if there is liable to be disturbance from or to adjacent spaces.
- Children's sensitivity to non high frequency fluorescent lamps should be checked with light fitting and hearing aid manufacturers[62].

It should be noted that the design of specialist accommodation for those with visual or hearing impairment is beyond the scope of this document and expert advice may be required.

B8 Designing for children and young people with mental health problems

A number of design issues that relate particularly to patients with mental health problems are covered throughout Section B. This section summarises the key design principles that relate to school facilities that will be used by patients with mental health problems, with particular reference to facilities that form part of a specialist mental health unit. In the case of such units, some spaces might be shared with the unit provision. For example a large space may be used for PE, music and drama as well as providing a social space (see Case Study 6).

- Ensure that the whole facility is fully secure with controlled locks (swipe cards, keypads etc.) and CCTV at entrances, and that outside areas are also fully secure.
- Provide a sense of safety and security without threat of intrusion. Ensure that all windows are secure and do not allow access either in or out (not allowing a patient to fall from or get through).

Notes

59 Note: All fabrics should comply with guidance in NHS Estates. **HFN 30. Infection control in the built environment.** TSO, 2002, and NHS Estates. **HTM 85: Fire precautions in existing hospitals.** HMSO, 1994, and **HTM 86: Fire risk assessment in hospitals.** HMSO, 1994.

60 Refer also to http://www.doh.gov.uk/dda/index.htm

61 See Department for Education and Skills. **Building Bulletin 93: Acoustic design of schools**, TSO (forthcoming, 2003) which includes advice on acoustic criteria for the hearing impaired. Draft available at http://www.teachernet.gov.uk/acoustics

62 The National Deaf Children Society (NDCS) state that designers should be aware that when some hearing aids are being used on the 'telecoil setting' (for example when an induction loop is being employed), electrical equipment, especially fluorescent light fittings, can sometimes cause interference. The problem occurs in situations where hearing aid wearers are close to the equipment (for example where there is a low ceiling).

- Ideally place the schoolroom close to, but clearly separate from, the associated mental health unit to identify this as an educational rather than treatment area.
- Make a calm, clear orderly layout of spaces, which give a positive and uplifting sense to the facility and allow easy navigation and orientation.
- Provide sufficient spaces to allow the full curriculum range to be covered including specialist facilities for science, design and technology and art (a minimum of appropriate materials, storage and a sink in the classroom for art).
- Ensure that pupils can have access to an alternative private space away from the main classroom area(s).
- Provide somewhere for pupils to do PE, either an activity room for key stage 1 and 2 or gym facilities.
- Ensure there is access to outside space including play areas for younger pupils.
- Ensure that rooms are spacious, light, airy and comfortable.
- Ensure that there is plenty of storage area, and that the furniture and equipment allows for well organised and efficient storage and retrieval so that the facility will feel calm and orderly.
- Ensure that any equipment or tools which are potentially harmful are secure: specify a lockable cupboard for classrooms (for scissors etc.) and a lockable cupboard for kitchens (knives etc.).
- Specify air hand dryers or paper towel dispensers in WCs rather than roller towels.
- Specify push-button/toggle rather than pull-cord electrical switches and alarm calls.

The key spatial characteristics of spaces designed for those with mental health problems is that they have a calm, orderly feel, too much colour or display in the classroom may be unsettling for some psychiatric patients. However, this needs to be balanced against the need to celebrate and encourage good work through display, common to all teaching/learning situations.

Section C: Case studies

The case studies are presented in four pages: **Data**, **Survey**, **Design advantages and disadvantages** and **Optimisation study**. The criteria for **optimisation** are based on the comments and observations made by teaching staff and pupils during the visit, and our own observations then and subsequently. In most cases we have kept to the existing area of each location, and rearranged the layout to accommodate the observed brief better. Obviously this is just one of many possible arrangements, and in many cases the resulting arrangements are not ideal in the sense that better provision could be provided in a new project. The intention is to provoke useful points of discussion for the design teams of future new and refurbished hospital schools.

Case study 1: Suite of classrooms in a large children's and young people's hospital

Data

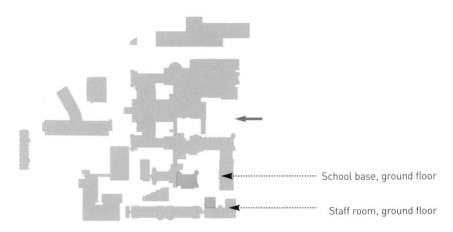

School base, ground floor

Staff room, ground floor

Type of hospital:	Tertiary referral hospital.
No. of childrens' beds in facility:	268 (plus small number of day patients).
Average stay for a pupil in hospital:	1 week to 2 years (on the psychiatric ward the average stay is about 10 months).
The hospital school:	The whole organisation, of which this example is a part, covers 11 sites, (of which 8 are hospitals), across the city. Home teaching is also offered where necessary. It is the largest home and hospital school service in Europe. The case study is one of the sites. It is designed as a suite and is located next to the paediatric wards.
Teaching area:	126m² (41%).
Non-teaching area:	183m² (59%).
Teaching area per pupil:	4.5m² (calculated on those in the school, not on the wards).
No. of planned places in school:	In the hospital school rooms, there are 16 places for secondary school pupils, plus 12 for primary level pupils. The school as a whole can cope with up to 176 pupils.
Typical number of pupils attending hospital school in a day:	Average approximately 148 in the school as a whole (28 in the school room and the rest on the wards).
Age range of pupils:	In theory 5-16 years (in practice 2-19 years).
Pupil medical need profile:	Majority of the pupils in the school rooms (60-70%) are from the psychiatric ward.
Staff in the hospital school:	12 FTE Teachers, 2.3 FTE Part Time Teachers, 6 Special School Assistants. 2 Part Time clerical (0.7 FTE).
Staff/pupil ratio:	1:8 (approximately).
Funding and ownership:	The hospital school building is owned by the NHS Trust; the school via the LEA pay a 'service charge' for maintenance and estate services.
Teaching accommodation:	The hospital school is part of the refurbished hospital building, (completed 1996-7). The design of the school was discussed in detail between the school staff, architects and the Trust from space requirements and layout down to finishes and colours. There are two dedicated classrooms, plus support areas. The majority of teaching is carried out on the wards.

Case study 1: Suite of classrooms in a large children's and young people's hospital

Survey

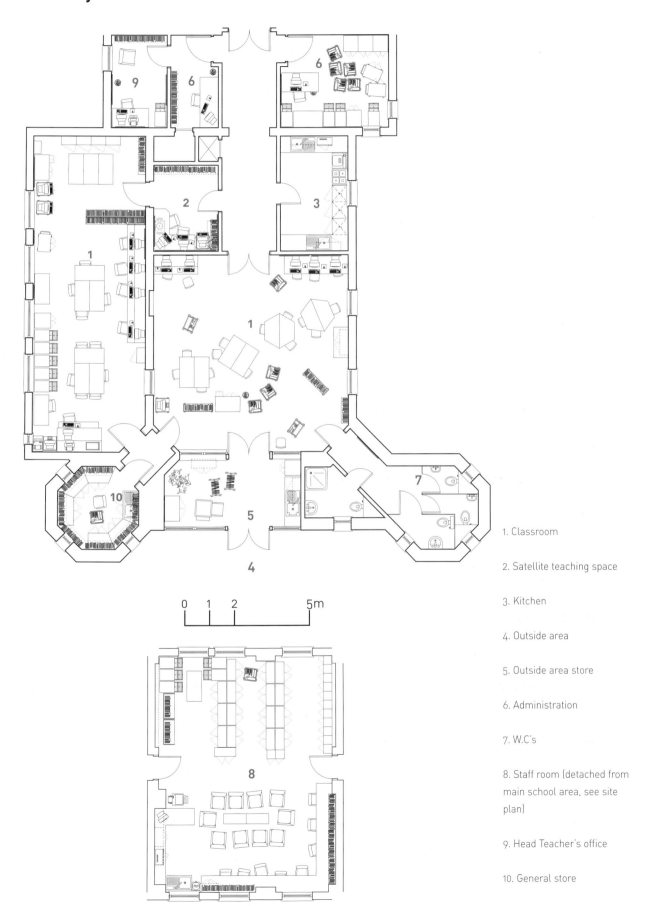

1. Classroom

2. Satellite teaching space

3. Kitchen

4. Outside area

5. Outside area store

6. Administration

7. W.C's

8. Staff room (detached from main school area, see site plan)

9. Head Teacher's office

10. General store

Case study 1: Suite of classrooms in a large children's and young people's hospital

Design advantages and disadvantages

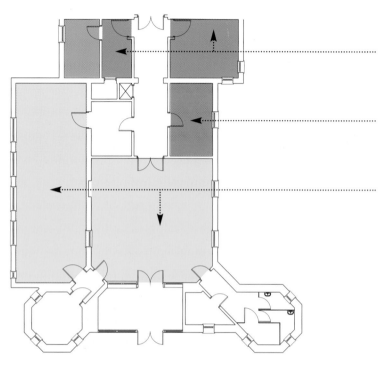

Design advantages

Separate offices for staff, plus administration office, and staff room, and head Teacher's office.

Kitchen for food technology and for staff use.

Good space provision: 2 separate classrooms for primary and secondary education, as well as a separate satellite teaching space (multi-media room, also used as an exam room, interview room and library).

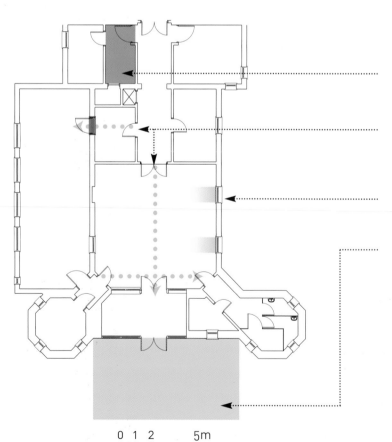

Design disadvantages

Not enough space for staff administration.

Poor circulation (need to pass through teaching areas to services). Doors not wide enough for beds.

Poor natural light (in primary schoolroom).

No designated, enclosed outdoor area, which is a security problem.

0 1 2   5m

Case study 1: Suite of classrooms in a large children's and young people's hospital

Optimisation study

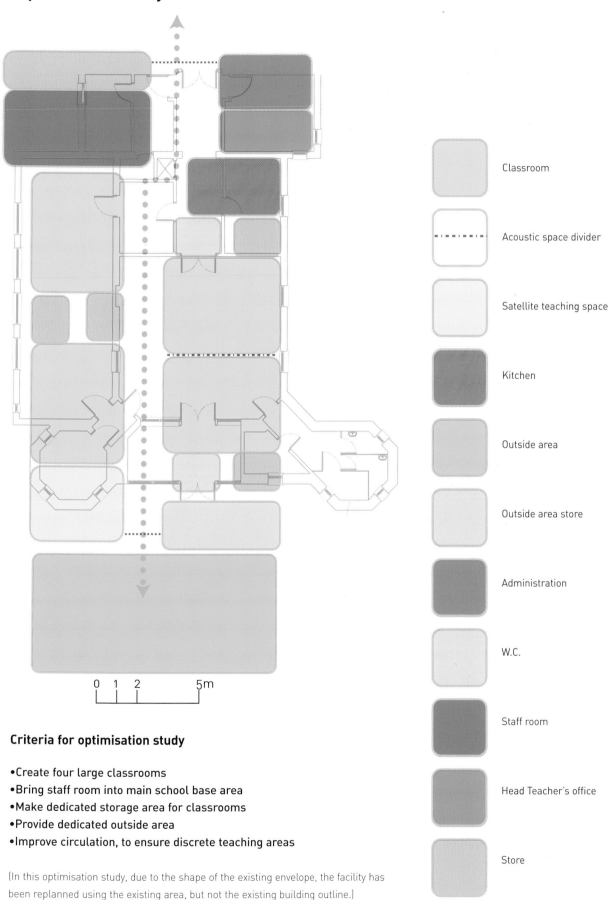

Classroom

Acoustic space divider

Satellite teaching space

Kitchen

Outside area

Outside area store

Administration

W.C.

Staff room

Head Teacher's office

Store

0 1 2   5m

Criteria for optimisation study

•Create four large classrooms
•Bring staff room into main school base area
•Make dedicated storage area for classrooms
•Provide dedicated outside area
•Improve circulation, to ensure discrete teaching areas

(In this optimisation study, due to the shape of the existing envelope, the facility has been replanned using the existing area, but not the existing building outline.)

Case study 2: Suite of classrooms in a specialist paediatric hospital

Data

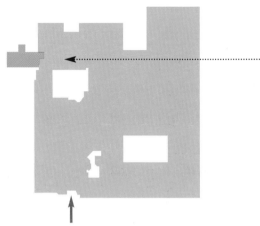

Hospital School, ground floor

Type of hospital:	Tertiary referral hospital.
No. of beds in facility:	360.
Average stay for a pupil in hospital:	From 1 week to several years continuously (most pupils stay a week, the average stay is two to three weeks).
The hospital school:	The school serves a specialist paediatric hospital.
Teaching area:	91m² (47%).
Non-teaching area:	104m² (53%).
Teaching area per pupil:	5.2m² (approximately).
No. of planned places in school:	123 planned places (including the classroom in the psychiatric ward) (See Case Study 6) on site and a general paediatric ward (off site) neither of which are drawn here).
Typical number of pupils attending schoolroom in a day:	Typically 15 to 20 (varies from 2 to 35). This number excludes the children taught on the wards and in the psychiatric unit. The school as a whole can teach up to 130 pupils.
Age range of pupils:	All school ages (i.e. 5-19 yrs) with a full range from A level to special needs.
Pupil medical need profile:	Mixed from all of the specialist ward areas of the hospital, which deals with a range of conditions.
Staff:	14 FTE Teachers, 5 FTE Teaching Assistants, 2 FTE support staff, 1 FTE senior administrative officer, I FTE general school helper (total 23 FTE).
Staff/pupil ratio:	1:6.
Funding and ownership:	The School is a foundation special school. It is funded through the LEA with mainly devolved capital.
Teaching accommodation:	The School currently occupies an adapted ward space. It has an outside courtyard, and is close to the play facility (adjacent). The planning of the space has resulted in all teaching (except for some ICT work) taking place in a single space, which is characteristically adapted several times over the course of a day to accommodate changes in demand.

Case study 2: Suite of classrooms in a specialist paediatric hospital

Survey

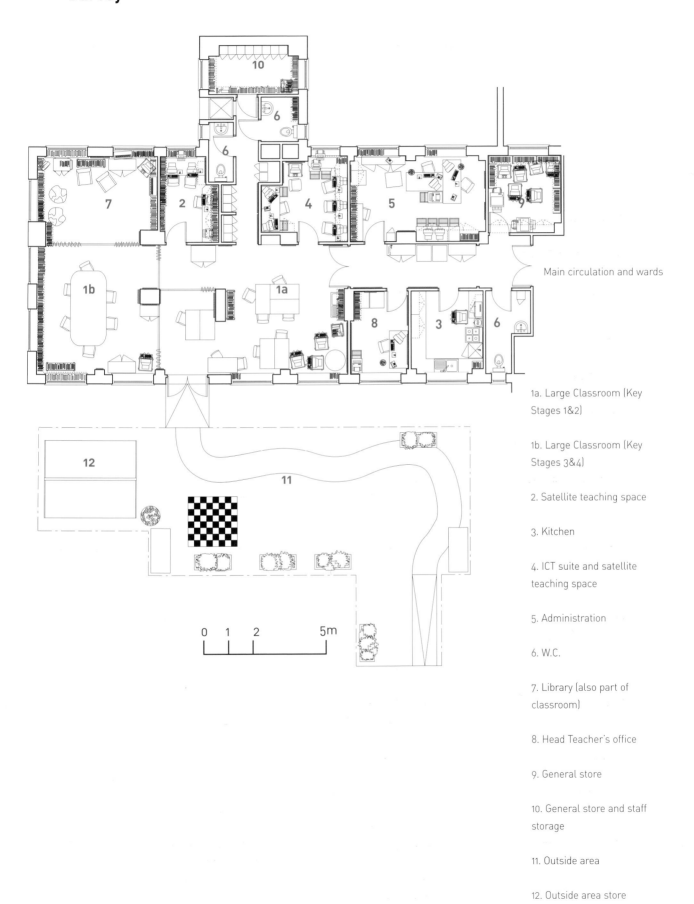

Main circulation and wards

1a. Large Classroom (Key Stages 1&2)

1b. Large Classroom (Key Stages 3&4)

2. Satellite teaching space

3. Kitchen

4. ICT suite and satellite teaching space

5. Administration

6. W.C.

7. Library (also part of classroom)

8. Head Teacher's office

9. General store

10. General store and staff storage

11. Outside area

12. Outside area store

Case study 2: Suite of classrooms in a specialist paediatric hospital

Design advantages and disadvantages

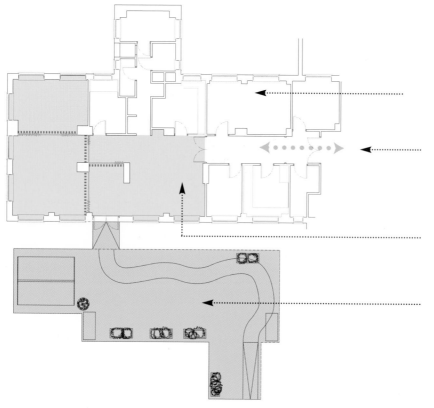

Design advantages

Reception/administration office close to entry.

Easy Access from the wards. Ground floor location ensures good visibility from hospital circulation route. Good security (swipe and CCTV).

A flexible, open plan and large classroom, divisible by curtains which can be opened up for group activities, P.E. etc.

Outside area accessible from the schoolroom.

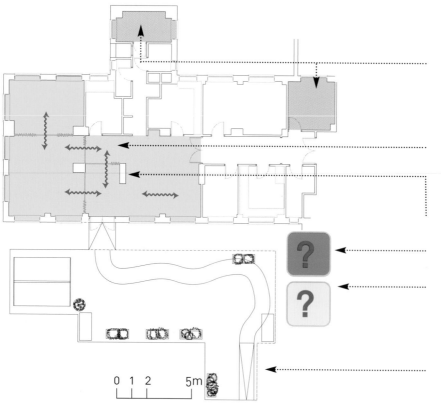

Design disadvantages

Insufficient storage space either for staff (personal belongings) or for storage of teaching material.

Classroom areas are separated by curtains only, so there is no sound isolation.

Structural pillars inhibit flexibility.

There is no staff room.

There is no separate space for teaching immune deficient children/taking exams/conducting interviews.

Weak point for security as it allows access to road.

0 1 2   5m

Case study 2: Suite of classrooms in a specialist paediatric hospital

Optimisation study

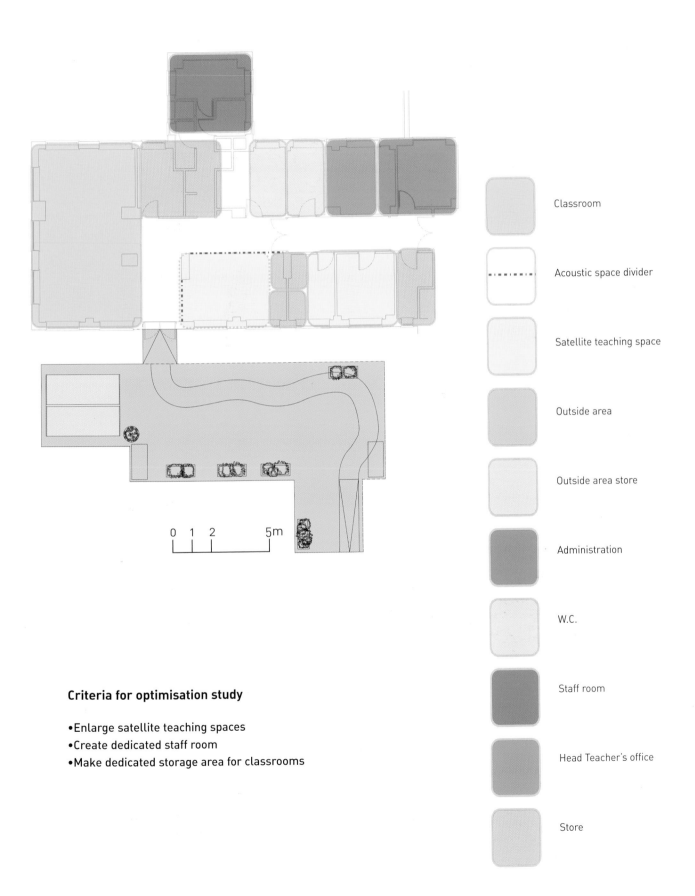

Classroom

Acoustic space divider

Satellite teaching space

Outside area

Outside area store

Administration

W.C.

Staff room

Head Teacher's office

Store

0 1 2   5m

Criteria for optimisation study

- Enlarge satellite teaching spaces
- Create dedicated staff room
- Make dedicated storage area for classrooms

Case study 3: Single schoolroom at a secondary referral hospital

Data

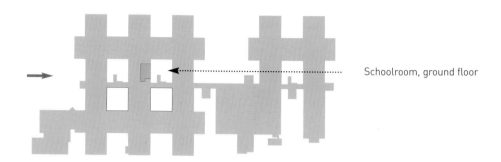

Schoolroom, ground floor

Type of hospital:	Secondary referral hospital.
No. of beds in facility:	22 beds in the children's ward (part of a general hospital).
Average stay for a pupil in hospital:	2 to 3 days (the shortest time is half a day, and the longest time is 6 to 8 weeks).
The hospital school:	One classroom located next to the paediatric wards and across the corridor from the Play Space.
Teaching area:	42.5m² (92%).
Non-teaching area:	3.5m² (8%).
Teaching area per pupil:	8.4m² (approximately).
No. of planned places in school unit:	10.
Typical number of pupils attending school unit in a day:	5 to 6.
Age range of pupils:	5 to 16 years (but will accommodate pupils outside of this range when necessary).
Pupil medical need profile:	85% physical illness, 15% mental illness.
Staff:	1.5 FTE Teachers, 1 FTE learning support assistant.
Staff/pupil ratio:	1:4.
Funding and ownership:	The School accommodation is owned by the NHS, who pay for all running costs. The LEA pays for all educational materials and for teaching staff.
Teaching accommodation:	Purpose built (although schoolroom and play space have been swapped to allow the play space access to an outdoor courtyard rather than the school).

Case study 3: Single schoolroom at a secondary referral hospital

Survey

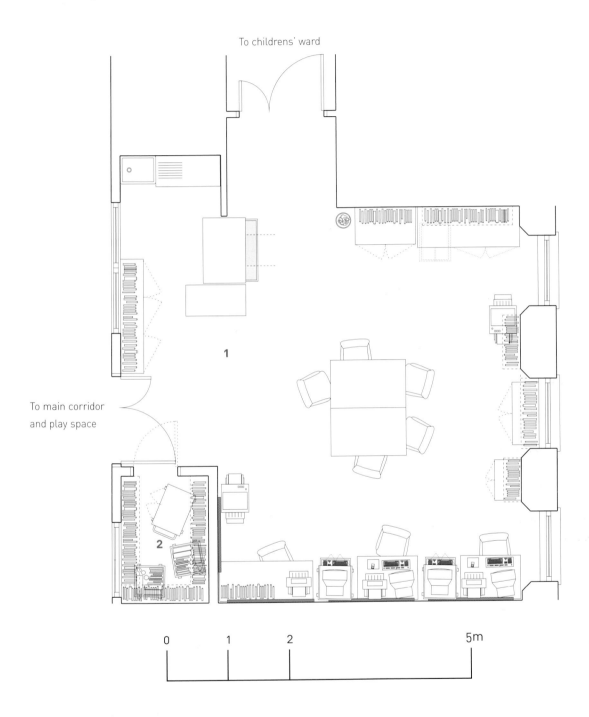

To childrens' ward

To main corridor
and play space

1

2

0 1 2 5m

1. Classroom

2. General store

Case study 3: Single schoolroom at a secondary referral hospital

Design advantages and disadvantages

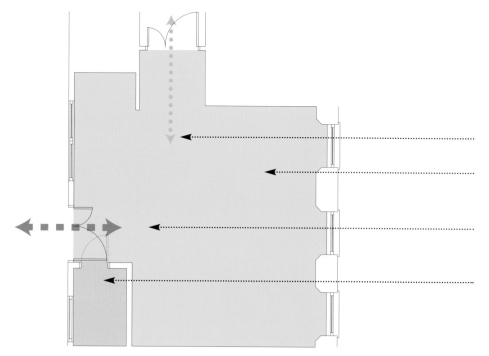

Design advantages

Good, direct access to ward.

Good size for school room.

Good access to play space (immediately opposite across corridor).

Dedicated storage for school room (though could usefully be larger).

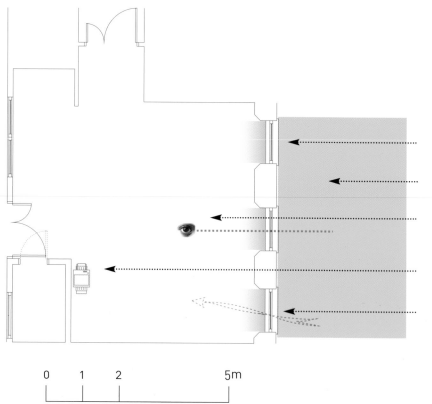

Design disadvantages

One-sided windows to outside gives poor daylight distribution.

No direct access to outside area.

Poor view out of school room.

School room is also used by medical staff (for example for photocopying).

Poor air quality and overheating resulting from no cross ventilation or adequate air-conditioning.

0   1   2   5m

Case study 3: Single schoolroom at a secondary referral hospital

Optimisation study

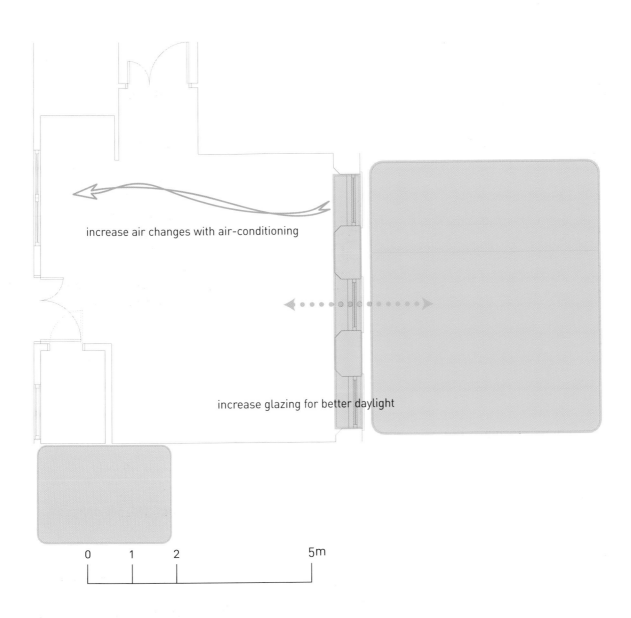

increase air changes with air-conditioning

increase glazing for better daylight

0   1   2   5m

Criteria for optimisation study

- Improve light distribution and increase air change rates
- Make access to dedicated outside space
- Increase dedicated storage area

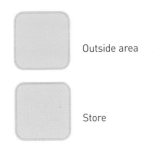

Outside area

Store

Case study 4: Suite of classrooms with satellite in a tertiary referral hospital

Data

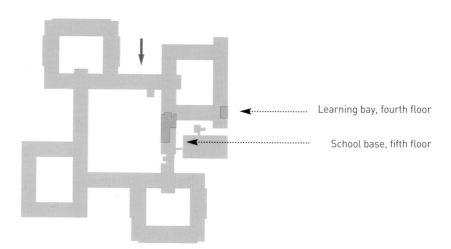

Learning bay, fourth floor

School base, fifth floor

Type of hospital:	A regional centre and tertiary referral hospital.
No. of beds in facility:	120.
Average stay for a pupil in hospital:	Ranges from half a day to 16 months (the average measured over a year is approximately 3 days).
The hospital school:	There are two areas in the hospital for teaching; the main hospital school (shown in the survey, and included in the above calculation) and a smaller 'learning bay' (shared with a play area) on a different level in a paediatric ward for orthopaedic patients (not shown in the survey but included in the area calculation).
Teaching area:	106m² (43%).
Non-teaching area:	140m² (57%).
Teaching area per pupil:	8.4m² (approximately).
No. of planned places in school:	45.
Typical number of pupils attending schoolroom in a day:	Approximately 30 (12-13 in the orthopaedic ward, and the remainder in the two classrooms of the main school). Note many pupils on the orthopaedic ward will be taught at the bedside.
Age range of pupils:	5 to 16+.
Pupil medical need profile:	The majority have physical illnesses and only a few have psychiatric illnesses.
Staff:	5 FTE Teachers. 1 FTE teaching support assistant. 0.5 clerical assistant.
Staff/pupil ratio:	1:5.
Funding and ownership:	The Hospital Trust owns the school accommodation but the LEA pay a rent per year which includes all services.
Teaching accommodation:	The main school area of 2 classrooms plus non-teaching areas and outdoor space was not purpose built, but the brief for educational need was taken into account when the adaptation was made. The learning zone on the orthopaedic ward is an adapted hospital bay.

Case study 4: Suite of classrooms with satellite in a tertiary referral hospital

Survey

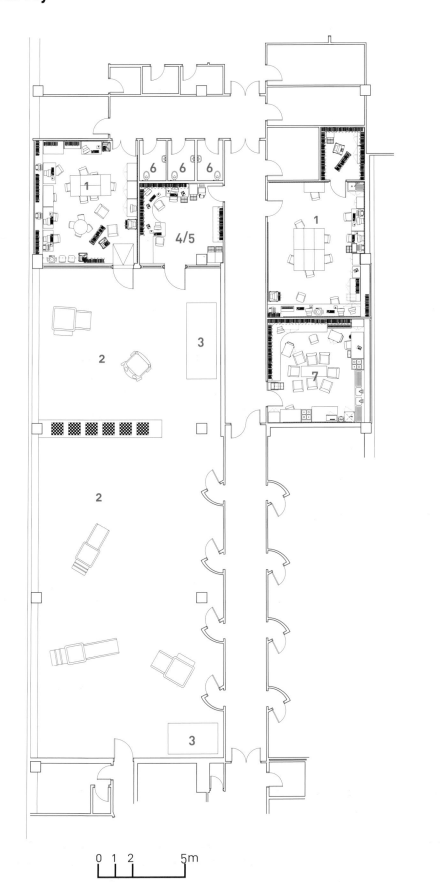

0 1 2   5m

1. Classroom

2. Outside area

3. Outside area store

4. Administration

5. Head Teacher's office

6. W.C.

7. Staff room

Case study 4: Suite of classrooms with satellite in a tertiary referral hospital

Design advantages and disadvantages

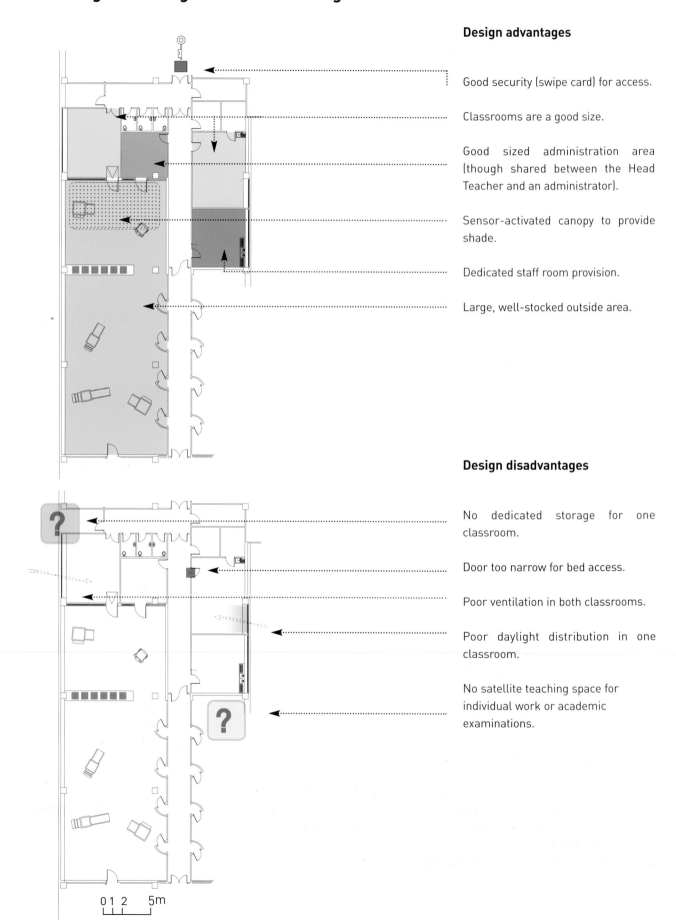

Design advantages

Good security (swipe card) for access.

Classrooms are a good size.

Good sized administration area (though shared between the Head Teacher and an administrator).

Sensor-activated canopy to provide shade.

Dedicated staff room provision.

Large, well-stocked outside area.

Design disadvantages

No dedicated storage for one classroom.

Door too narrow for bed access.

Poor ventilation in both classrooms.

Poor daylight distribution in one classroom.

No satellite teaching space for individual work or academic examinations.

0 1 2   5m

Case study 4: Suite of classrooms with satellite in a tertiary referral hospital

Optimisation study

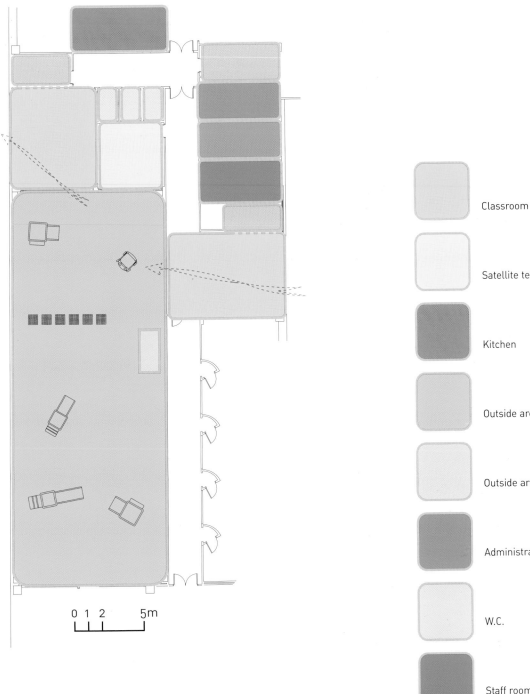

0 1 2   5m

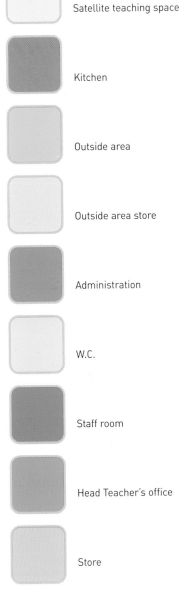

Classroom

Satellite teaching space

Kitchen

Outside area

Outside area store

Administration

W.C.

Staff room

Head Teacher's office

Store

Criteria for optimisation study

•Improve light distribution and allow cross-ventilation in classroom by increasing window proportion and having windows on two elevations
•Make a satellite teaching space (to allow quiet study, for example, for older pupils)
•Make dedicated storage area for both classooms

Case study 5: Young people's unit in a tertiary referral hospital

Data

Childrens' ward schoolroom, sixth floor

Adolescent unit, first floor floor

Oncology ward schoolroom, second floor

Type of hospital:	Tertiary referral hospital.
No. of beds in facility:	19 in the young people's unit, 10 in the oncology ward. 13 in the children's ward.
Average stay for a pupil in hospital (all ages):	75% stay between 1 and 4 weeks or have a recurrent illness.
The hospital school:	There are three distinct areas for teaching children and young people: a children's ward with a very small dedicated classroom, a small bay in the young people's cancer ward, and a purpose built young people's unit. All of the spaces are used in the area calculations, but only the young people's unit is included as a drawn survey.
Teaching area:	50m^2 (81%).
Non-teaching area:	12m^2 (19%).
Teaching area per pupil:	5.5m^2 approximately (with an average of about nine pupils in the two schoolrooms).
No. of planned places in school:	10 in the young people's unit, 2 in the oncology ward, 4 in the children's ward.
Typical number of pupils attending school in a day:	Approximately 15 in all designated teaching areas including the wards (2-4 children in the childrens' ward schoolroom, 1-6 pupils in the young people's ward and in the oncology ward teaching is carried out almost exclusively at the bedside).
Age range of pupils (adolescent unit):	14-19.
Pupil medical need profile (all ages):	Patients all have life threatening or chronic illnesses.
Staff:	5 FTE Teachers and 1 youth worker (for all areas), 0.25 FTE clerical support.
Staff/pupil ratio:	1:4.
Funding and ownership:	The educational facility is owned by the Trust who also pay running costs (heating and lighting). The LEA pays for telephone, teaching and materials.
Teaching accommodation:	A purpose built young people's unit comprising: a resource base and teachers' office. There are associated spaces which are part of the unit, but not directly controlled by the facility, including a youth worker's office, a seminar room, staff room, kitchen and a social area. The oncology ward has a corner with space for a computer which is used as a teaching space. The children's ward has a small schoolroom.

Case study 5: Young people's unit in a tertiary referral hospital

Survey

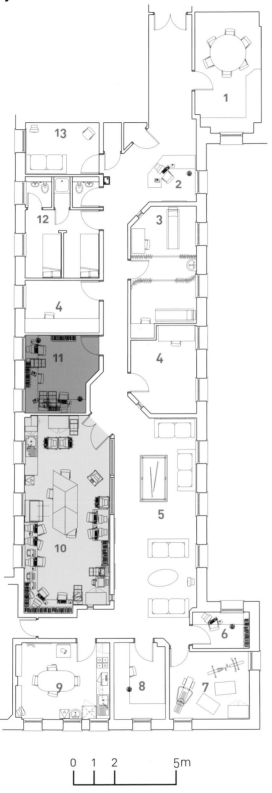

0   1   2   5m

1. Doctor/Team meeting
   room

2. Unit reception

3. Medical examination room

4. Medical interview room

5. Recreational area

6. Youth Worker's office

7. Exercise room

8. Craft room

9. Kitchen

10. Classroom

11. Teachers' office

12. Parents' accommodation

13. Parents' quiet room

Coloured areas indicate core
educational rooms.

Note: The Adolescent Unit is set up on a principle of teamworking
between educational, medical and other professionals, which means
that all spaces within the unit are shared to a greater or lesser extent
as required. This gives greater flexibility to the educational facility, for
example use of interview rooms for exams or quiet study.

Case study 5: Young people's unit in a tertiary referral hospital

Design advantages and disadvantages

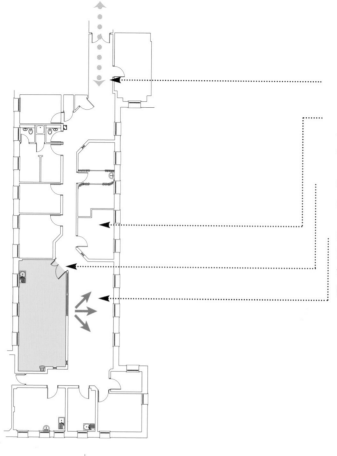

Design advantages

Good access to ward.

Medical rooms occasionally made available for educational purposes such as academic examinations.

Classroom can be shut off from socialising and medical areas.

Good connections to social space (snooker, relaxing), kitchen (snacks for parents, and made by parents for patients), exercise room (for physio) etc.

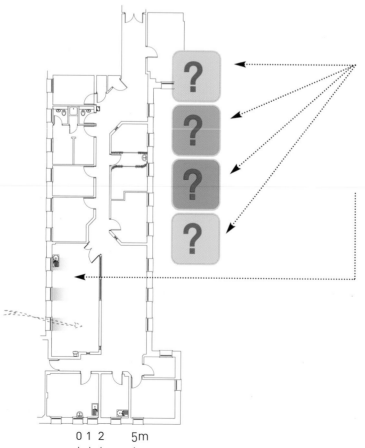

Design disadvantages

No dedicated head teacher's office, administration room, store, or adjacent outside area (though these disadvantages are partially mitigated by the sharing space philosophy that underpins the unit).

Poor ventilation and daylight to resource base, which is an awkward, long, thin shape.

0 1 2   5m

Case study 5: Young people's unit in a tertiary referral hospital

Optimisation study

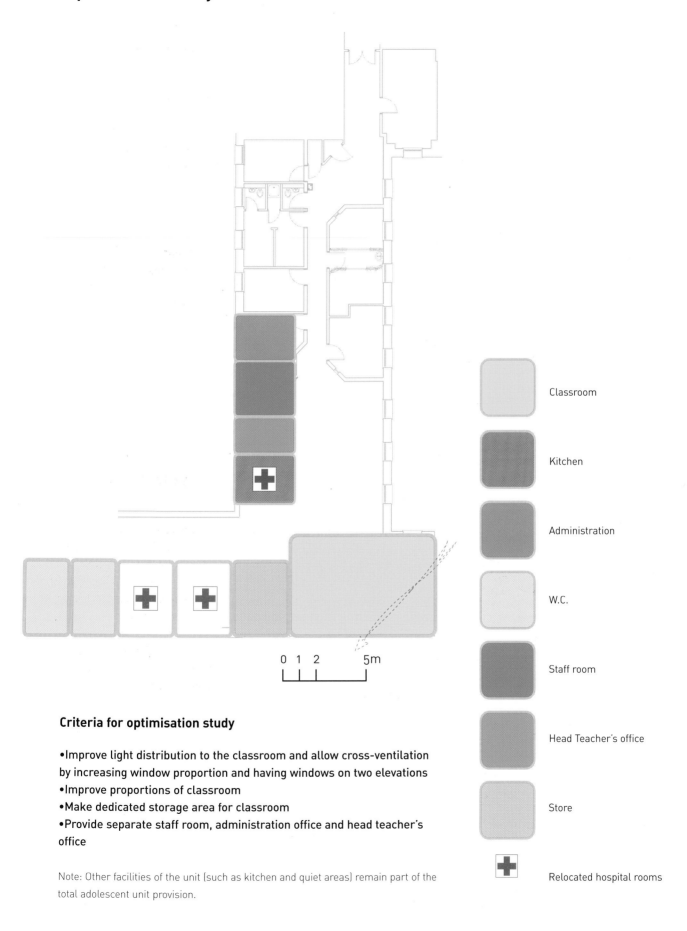

Classroom

Kitchen

Administration

W.C.

Staff room

Head Teacher's office

Store

Relocated hospital rooms

0 1 2   5m

Criteria for optimisation study

•Improve light distribution to the classroom and allow cross-ventilation by increasing window proportion and having windows on two elevations
•Improve proportions of classroom
•Make dedicated storage area for classroom
•Provide separate staff room, administration office and head teacher's office

Note: Other facilities of the unit (such as kitchen and quiet areas) remain part of the total adolescent unit provision.

Case study 6: Psychiatric unit in a tertiary referral hospital

Data

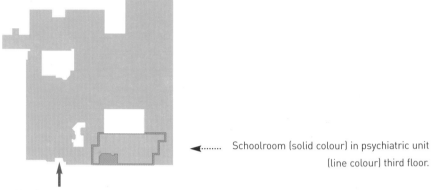

⯇........ Schoolroom (solid colour) in psychiatric unit
(line colour) third floor.

Type of hospital:	Tertiary referral hospital.
No. of beds in the facility:	10.
Average stay for a pupil in the facility:	Typically 4 months, but this varies between a 6 week assessment and one year plus. Some pupils are re-admitted if a relapse occurs.
The hospital school:	The school serves a specialist psychiatric unit for children and young people. The facility is situated within the main hospital but has separate accommodation and schoolroom for patients.
Teaching area:	32m² (100%).
Non-teaching area:	Supported from main school (see Case study 2).
Teaching area per pupil:	5.3m².
No. of planned places in school:	10.
Typical number of pupils attending school in a day:	6.
Age range of pupils:	7-16 years.
Pupil medical need profile:	Pupils are all referred due to psychiatric illnesses and related problems.
Staff:	Staff are allocated from the main hospital school, (see Case study 2). These are 1 FTE and 3 part time teachers (0.6 FTE combined total), plus one full time teaching assistant.
Staff/pupil ratio:	1:3 (approximately).
Funding and ownership:	The educational facility is owned by the Trust who also pay running costs (heating and lighting). The Foundation School pays a peppercorn rent and for cleaning, telephone, teaching and materials.
Teaching accommodation:	The school comprises one classroom. Within the facility, a large central space sub-divided with curtains, (which the classroom gives onto), can occasionally be used for 1:1 teaching for pupils who are not able to work in the classroom, and also for music and dance. The main hospital school is also used for several teaching lessons a week which is part of an inclusive approach. All support teaching spaces are located in the main hospital school (Case study 2).

Case study 6: Psychiatric unit in a tertiary referral hospital

Survey

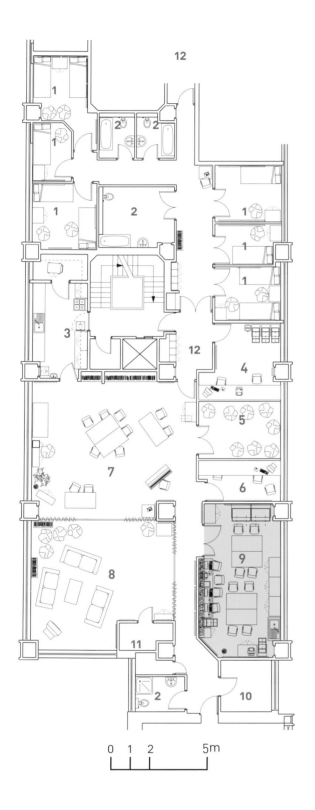

0 1 2 5m

1. Bedroom

2. Bathroom/W.C

3. Kitchen

4. Main Office

5. Treatment Room

6. Office

7. Dining Area

8. Living/TV area

9. Classroom

10. Utility

11. Store

12. Entrance to Unit

Note: The classroom is located within the psychiatric unit, and some
sharing of other spaces (such as the Dining and Living/TV area, and the small
office adjacent) takes place. The area dedicated for classroom use only is coloured.
Staff and resources are supplied from the School base (see Case Study 2).

Case study 6: Psychiatric unit in a tertiary referral hospital

Design advantages and disadvantages

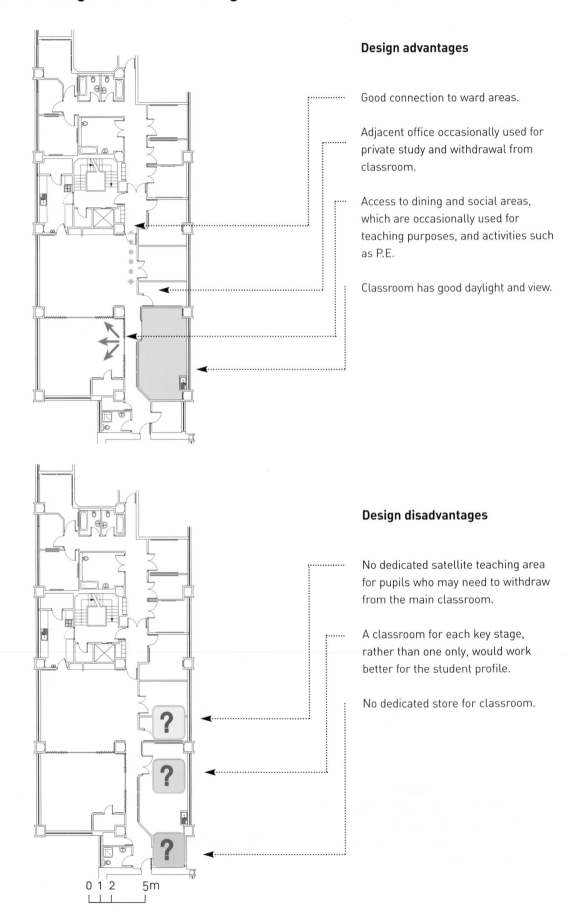

Design advantages

Good connection to ward areas.

Adjacent office occasionally used for private study and withdrawal from classroom.

Access to dining and social areas, which are occasionally used for teaching purposes, and activities such as P.E.

Classroom has good daylight and view.

Design disadvantages

No dedicated satellite teaching area for pupils who may need to withdraw from the main classroom.

A classroom for each key stage, rather than one only, would work better for the student profile.

No dedicated store for classroom.

0 1 2   5m

Case study 6: Psychiatric unit in a tertiary referral hospital

Optimisation study

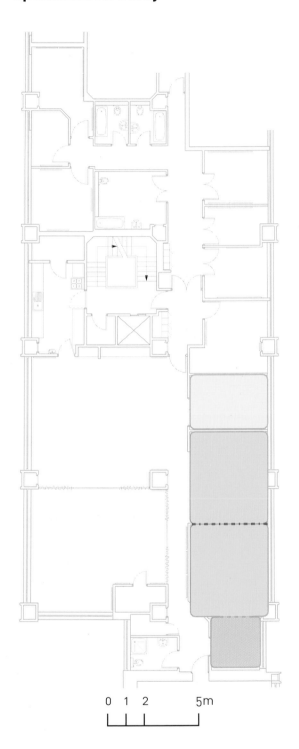

0 1 2 5m

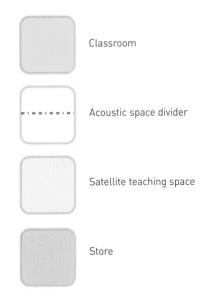

Classroom

Acoustic space divider

Satellite teaching space

Store

Criteria for optimisation study

•Make separate classrooms for two key stages, and allow for a large space to be made by combining these
•Make dedicated storage area for classroom
•Provide a satellite teaching space for pupils who may need to withdraw or for private study

Case study 7: School attached to psychiatric unit for young people

Data

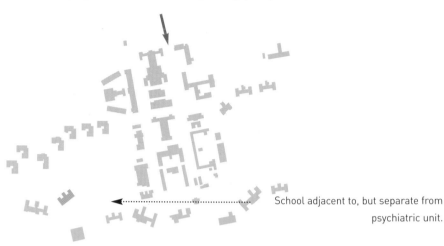

School adjacent to, but separate from psychiatric unit.

Type of facility:	The unit shares a large site with other units accommodating adults with learning difficulties.
No. of beds in the unit:	14.
Average stay for a pupil in the unit:	9 months (approximately).
The school:	A school in a psychiatric unit for young people within the fourth tier in CAMHS (Child Adolescent Mental Health Service).
Teaching area:	80.6m² (32%).
Non-teaching area:	174.8m² (68%).
Teaching area per pupil:	10m².
No. of planned places in school:	14.
Typical number of pupils attending school in a day:	8 (remaining 6 on roll will be taught in unit or being taken through reintegration into mainstream school).
Age range of pupils:	12-17 years.
Pupil medical need profile:	Pupils are all referred due to psychiatric illnesses and related problems.
Staff:	3 FTE teachers and 0.6 FTE secretarial/classroom assistant.
Staff/pupil ratio:	1:4 (approximately).
Funding and ownership:	The educational facility is owned by the Hospital Trust who also pay running costs (heating and lighting). The LEA pays for all internal resources and teachers.
Teaching accommodation:	The school comprises: 3 teaching rooms, (a main classroom, a music room and an art room), a main hall, a shared hall, Head Teacher's office, staff room, secretary's room and a kitchen. The pupils and staff have built a pond and planted an orchard in the surrounding grounds which they also use for games and recreation.

Case study 7: School attached to psychiatric unit for young people

Survey

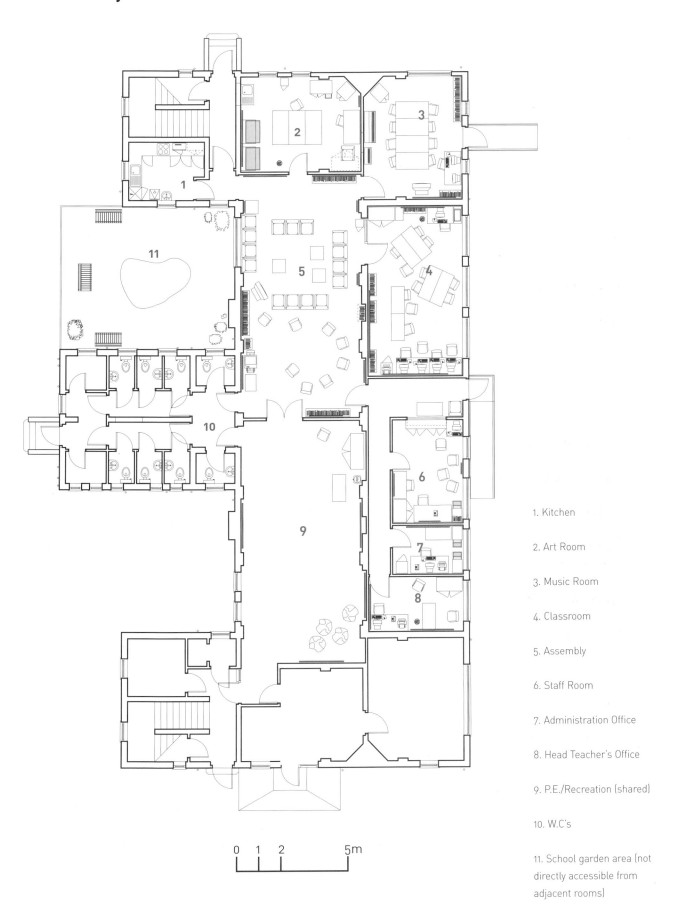

1. Kitchen

2. Art Room

3. Music Room

4. Classroom

5. Assembly

6. Staff Room

7. Administration Office

8. Head Teacher's Office

9. P.E./Recreation (shared)

10. W.C's

11. School garden area (not directly accessible from adjacent rooms)

0 1 2 5m

Case study 7: School attached to psychiatric unit for young people

Design advantages and disadvantages

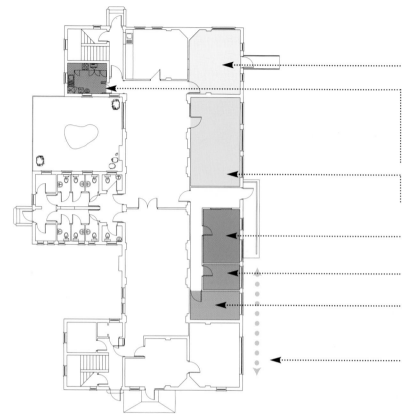

Design advantages

Satellite teaching space useful for pupils who need to withdraw from main classroom, and for music lessons (could usefully double as language facility).

Kitchen, can be used for teaching.

Well proportioned, light classroom.

Dedicated staff room.

Dedicated administration office.

Dedicated Head Teachers' office.

Good access to adjacent psychiatric unit, while maintaining important separation for school.

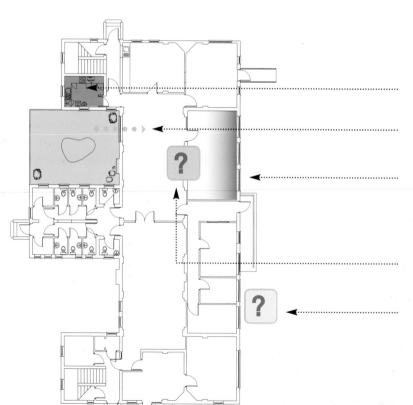

Design disadvantages

Kitchen is large enough for one or two pupils only.

Outdoor space is not fully secure, nor accessible directly from the school.

Classroom window orientation causes glare and reflection problems for screens and whiteboard, and overheating in summer.

Classroom does not have dedicated store.

No dedicated design and technology area.

0 1 2   5m

Case study 7: School attached to psychiatric unit for young people

Optimisation study

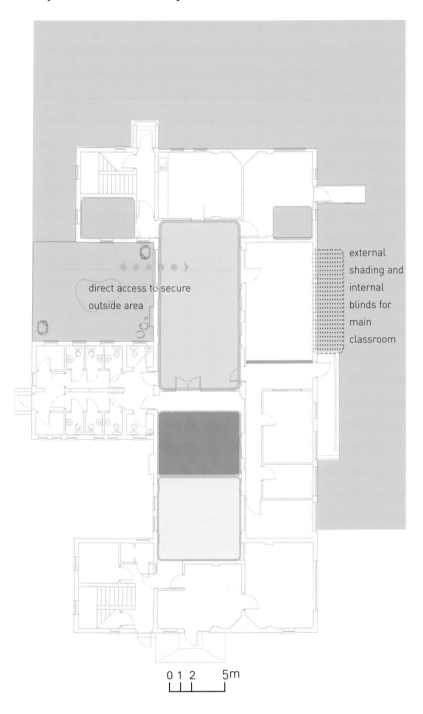

direct access to secure outside area

external shading and internal blinds for main classroom

0 1 2   5m

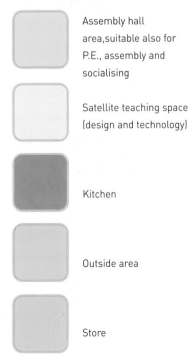

Assembly hall area, suitable also for P.E., assembly and socialising

Satellite teaching space (design and technology)

Kitchen

Outside area

Store

Criteria for optimisation study

- Create a general store and dedicated storage for classroom
- Add external shading and internal blinds for classroom
- Create a larger kitchen
- Create dedicated design and technology area (this is a request of the School, which considers that this would be a useful facility, particularly suited to the pupil profile)
- Convert assembly hall area for more varied use, including P.E., drama and social events
- Create a dedicated, secure outside area

Key to symbols

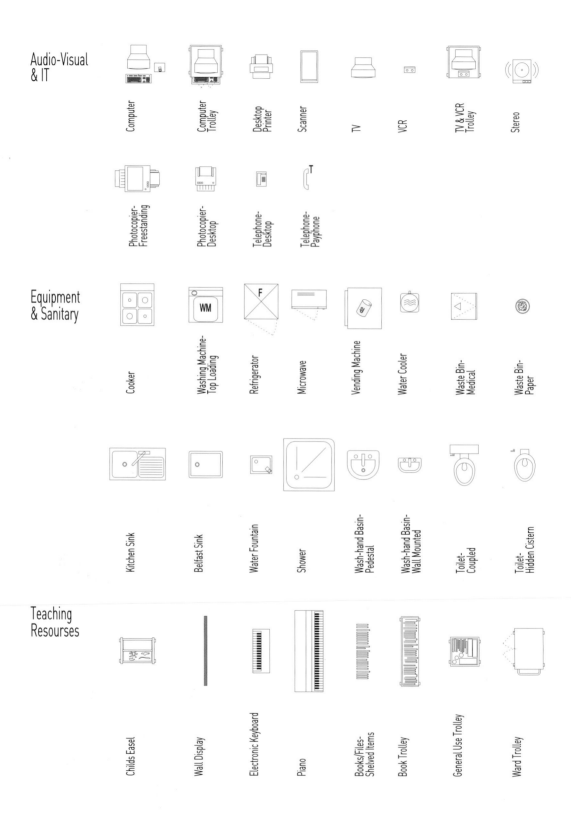

Audio-Visual & IT

Computer

Computer Trolley

Desktop Printer

Scanner

TV

VCR

TV & VCR Trolley

Stereo

Photocopier-Freestanding

Photocopier-Desktop

Telephone-Desktop

Telephone-Payphone

Equipment & Sanitary

Cooker

Washing Machine-Top Loading

Refrigerator

Microwave

Vending Machine

Water Cooler

Waste Bin-Medical

Waste Bin-Paper

Kitchen Sink

Belfast Sink

Water Fountain

Shower

Wash-hand Basin-Pedestal

Wash-hand Basin-Wall Mounted

Toilet-Coupled

Toilet-Hidden Cistern

Teaching Resourses

Childs Easel

Wall Display

Electronic Keyboard

Piano

Books/Files-Shelved Items

Book Trolley

General Use Trolley

Ward Trolley

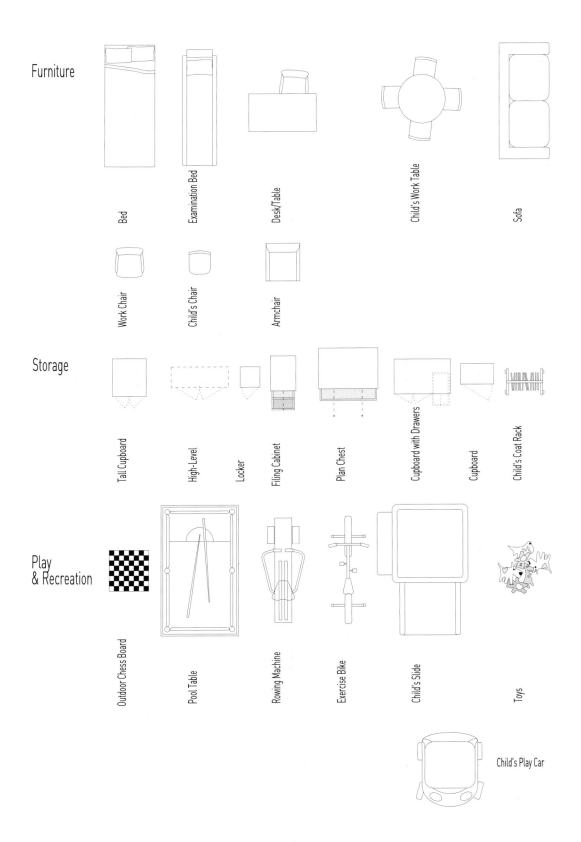

Furniture

Bed

Examination Bed

Desk/Table

Child's Work Table

Sofa

Work Chair

Child's Chair

Armchair

Storage

Tall Cupboard

High-Level

Locker

Filing Cabinet

Plan Chest

Cupboard with Drawers

Cupboard

Child's Coat Rack

Play & Recreation

Outdoor Chess Board

Pool Table

Rowing Machine

Exercise Bike

Child's Slide

Toys

Child's Play Car

Glossary and acronyms

AEDET: The "Achieving Excellence Design Evaluation Toolkit" published by the NHS Estates for hospital design.

Barrier Nursing: Patient nursed in isolation because of infection which may be contagious. Equipment for use with such patients must be disposable or washable and be thoroughly disinfected before being returned to normal use.

CCTV: Closed circuit television, generally used for visual surveillance.

CD-ROM: Compact Disk Read Only Memory.

DDA: Disability Discrimination Act.

Design and Technology: National Curriculum subject area which involves pupils in designing and making in a range of materials.

Duration of stay: Period spent by a patient for a single admission event.

DRC: Disability Rights Commission.

Dialysis: Artificial filtering of the blood outside the body, to compensate for kidney malfunction.

Food Technology: Part of design and technology where pupils work with food.

FTE: Full Time Equivalent.

Glare: The discomfort or impairment of vision experienced when parts of the visual field are excessively bright in relation to the general surroundings.

Home School: The school where a pupil may have been enrolled before entering hospital and/or to which they may go after leaving hospital.

Hospital Trust: The management body for a hospital.

ICT: Information Communication and Technology.

Key Stage (KS): The statutory school years are divided into four phases which mark stages of development. These approximate to ages as follows: beginning of compulsory education to age 7 (KS1); age 7-11 (KS2); age 11-14 (KS3); and age 14 to end of compulsory education (KS4).

LEA: Local Education Authority.

Lux: A measurement of illuminance (the amount of light falling on a given surface in lumens per metre squared).

National Curriculum: Statutory framework for specifying the content of the curriculum common between all schools.

Neutropaenic: Immune deficient.

NHS: National Health Service.

NSF: National Service Framework - Department of Health.

Oncology: Relating to the treatment of cancer.

Orthopaedic: Relating to the correction of bone injuries or deformities.

Play Specialist: Trained person designated to working with and supporting children.

Psychiatric: Relating to mental disorder.

Psychological: Relating to the functioning of the mind.

Psychosomatic: Relating to disease exacerbated by worry.

Renal: Relating to the kidneys.

Reverse Barrier Nursing: Patient nursed in isolation to prevent infection (for example, of an open wound, scald, burn). Equipment for use with such patients may be washed in disinfectant before being used, or may need to be new on each occasion.

SEN: Special Educational Needs.

Teamworking: Cross-disciplinary working practice between clinical, educational and other key professionals designed to deliver the best all round care for the patient.

Therapeutic: Pertaining to the physical or psychological amelioration of a condition.

Video conferencing: The linking of two or more users via web cams to facilitate real time interaction and communication with images.

Web-cam: A digital image camera linked directly to a computer capable of real time transmission of moving images.

Work Plan: The plan of tasks specific to each pupil in each of their subject areas.

Youth Worker: Trained person designated to working with and supporting young people.

Index

A

acoustic separation, 42, 48, 49

administrative office, 8, 12, 14, 18, 27, 28

anaemia, 47

B

beds, 8, 9, 18, 28, 30, 31, 35

blinds, 36, 44, 45, 46

C

CCTV, 20, 27, 49

ceilings, 34, 35, 44, 49

chemotherapy, 10, 32

circulation, 28, 30, 43, 44

colour, 36, 44, 46, 50

consultation, 8

corridors, 30, 39, 40, 43, 46

creative arts, 11, 14

cystic fibrosis, 24

D

dehydration, 47

design and technology, 11, 21, 50

Disability Discrimination Act, 12

Disability Rights Commission Act, 12

dialysis, 10

display, 3, 34, 38, 40, 41, 42, 50

doors, 35

drama, 8, 14, 30, 42, 44, 49

E

entrance areas, 27, 28

F

food technology, 29

fundraising, 30

furniture, 21, 26, 36, 37, 38, 39, 40, 50

G

gardening, 32

glare, 44, 45, 46

H

hearing impairment, 49

Home School, 7, 15, 26, 25

Hospital Trust, 4, 7, 18, 20, 28, 29

I

ICT, 4, 15, 16, 25, 39, 46, 47

infection control, 34, 42, 45

immune deficient, 10, 18, 25

isolation teaching, 10, 15, 25, 26

K

kitchens, 29, 37

L

lighting, 36, 43, 44, 45, 46

Local Education Authority, 1, 4, 6, 7, 8, 25

lux, 43

M

means of escape, 20, 40, 44, 46

mental health problems, 1, 4, 9, 11, 13, 22, 29, 34, 49, 50

music, 14, 24, 30, 42, 49

N

National Curriculum, 6, 13

National Service Framework, 1, 7

neutropaenic, 10

O

oncology, 24

outside space, 11, 18, 19, 30, 32, 49

P

parents, 12, 18, 20, 27, 28, 47

partitions, 42, 49

PE, 11, 13, 30, 49, 50

play specialist, 8, 12, 13, 16

psychiatric, 11, 21, 50

S

safety glass, 34, 35

science, 11, 13, 50

security, 11, 18, 20, 27, 33, 35, 39, 49

SEN, 9, 12, 15, 47

shade, 32, 45

shelving, 27, 40, 41

siblings, 12

staff room, 8, 18, 24, 27, 28

T

tables, 22, 36, 38, 39

teamworking, 8

textiles, 34

toilets, 20, 29, 34

V

vision panels, 35

visual impairment, 4, 45, 46, 49

W

walls, 34, 38, 49

ward teaching, 10, 13, 14, 24, 25, 26, 41

web-cam, 16

wheelchair, 9, 22, 29, 32, 35, 37

windows, 35, 36, 40, 45, 46, 47, 48, 49

work plan, 10, 15, 16

Y

youth worker, 8, 12, 16, 28